The Insomnia Breakthrough:

Effective Strategies to Fall Asleep, Sleep Through the Night, and Wake Feeling Refreshed

Katherine Coleman, LMT

Copyright © 2024 Katherine Coleman, LMT. All rights reserved.

The content of this book may not be reproduced, duplicated, or transmitted without direct written permission from the author or the publisher.

Under no circumstances will any blame or legal responsibility be held against the publisher or author for any damages, reparation, or monetary loss due to the information contained within this book. Either directly or indirectly. You are responsible for your own choices, actions, and results.

Legal Notice: This book is copyright-protected. This book is only for personal use. You cannot amend, distribute, sell, use, quote, or paraphrase any part or the content within this book without the author's or publisher's consent.

Disclaimer Notice:

Please note the information contained within this document is for educational and entertainment purposes only. All effort has been executed to present accurate, up-to-date, and reliable, complete information. No warranties of any kind are declared or implied. Readers acknowledge that the author is not engaging in the rendering of legal, financial, medical, or professional advice. The content within this book has been derived from various sources. Please consult a licensed professional before attempting any techniques outlined in this book.

By reading this document, the reader agrees that the author is under no circumstances responsible for any losses and/or damages, direct or indirect, incurred as a result of using the information contained within this document, including, but not limited to, errors, omissions, or inaccuracies.

Contents

Introduction	1
1. Understanding Insomnia and Its Impact	3
2. Psychological Triggers of Insomnia	14
3. Lifestyle and Environmental Adjustments	26
4. Diet, Exercise, and Sleep	40
5. Mindfulness and Relaxation Techniques	53
6. Cognitive Behavioral Therapy for Insomnia (CBT-I)	65
7. Special Considerations in Insomnia Management	77
8. Advanced Techniques and Therapies	90
9. Building Resilience and Maintaining Sleep Health	105
10. Future Trends and Innovations in Sleep Science	120
Conclusion	129
References	131

Introduction

Every night, countless individuals lie in bed, staring at the ceiling in silent frustration. You may know the feeling all too well—the desperate yearning for sleep that just won't come. It's not just you; millions share this nightly struggle. This isn't merely about missing a few hours of rest; it's about seeking liberation from the relentless grip of insomnia.

My journey into the world of sleep began not in a lab, but in my own life and the lives of my clients. I was both a witness and a participant in the elusive chase for a good night's sleep. This personal and professional connection drove me to dive deeper, transforming my curiosity into a dedicated pursuit of knowledge. Today, I stand before you not just as an observer, but as someone who has lived through the very experiences I write about. This book is the culmination of years of in-depth exploration, enriched by my hands-on experiences and strengthened by my exposure to my client's battles with insomnia.

"The Insomnia Breakthrough" is designed to be your guide through the often misunderstood landscape of insomnia. Here, we break down complex scientific concepts into practical, actionable steps. This book is committed to providing a clear path to understanding your sleep patterns and, more importantly, restoring them.

Drawing on a wealth of research, personal experiences, and extensive work with my clients, I offer you not just theories, but proven strategies. They are backed by science, yet they are explained here with the simplicity and clarity you need to make meaningful changes in your life.

This isn't just another collection of sleep advice. It's a different approach—synthesizing personal insights, scientific data, and practical solutions tailored to help you reclaim the restful sleep you deserve. Throughout these pages, you will find not only information but also inspiration. This book covers everything from understanding the root causes of insomnia to implementing daily routines that promote healthy sleep.

You are far from alone in this struggle. Current research shows that a significant portion of the global population battles with some form of sleep disruption. This book acknowledges and addresses the widespread nature of the issue, offering solace and solutions.

By the time you turn the final page, you'll have gained a deeper understanding of what causes sleep difficulties and how to overcome them. You'll learn new, healthier sleep practices and feel empowered to implement the changes leading to better sleep.

I invite you to join me with an open mind and a readiness to try new strategies. Let this book help you on a transformative journey toward nights filled with peaceful, uninterrupted sleep. There is hope, and it starts here, with your decision to take this vital step towards improving your life through better sleep.

Together, let's break through the barriers of insomnia and greet each morning refreshed, revitalized, and eager to embrace the day.

Chapter One

Understanding Insomnia and Its Impact

Defining Insomnia: More Than Just Sleeplessness

Have you ever spent the night tossing and turning, haunted by the ticking clock that seemed to echo louder with each passing minute? If so, you're not alone. Across the globe, millions find themselves caught in the frustrating cycle of insomnia, struggling not just to fall asleep, but to stay asleep or to wake too early without being able to drift back into slumber. This chapter seeks to peel back the layers of this prevalent condition, offering clarity and shedding light on the often misunderstood nuances of insomnia.

What is Insomnia

Insomnia is commonly believed to be the inability to fall asleep. However, its definition in the clinical sense is broader and more encompassing. Insomnia includes difficulty falling asleep, staying asleep, or waking up too early and unable to fall asleep again. The American Academy of Sleep Medicine defines insomnia as a disorder where individuals have trouble sleeping despite having the chance to do so. This difficulty can lead to functional impairment while awake and can occur despite adequate opportunities and circumstances for sleep.

It's crucial to differentiate between the perception and the reality of insomnia. Many individuals believe they suffer from insomnia if they do not achieve eight hours of sleep, adhering to the longstanding myth that this is the required amount for all adults. However, sleep needs vary across individuals, and insomnia depends more on the quality of sleep and how one feels during the day. This subjective nature means that even if you spend sufficient hours asleep, you might still feel exhausted if the sleep quality is poor. This distinction is vital because it emphasizes that insomnia can be as much about the perception of non-restorative sleep as it is about quantifiable sleep hours.

Understanding and practicing good sleep hygiene is critical to effectively tackling insomnia. Sleep hygiene refers to the behaviors and environmental factors that precisely influence our ability to sleep well. Unfortunately, poor sleep habits are often ingrained in our routines, whether scrolling through smartphones before bedtime, consuming caffeine late in the day, or having irregular sleep schedules. These habits can significantly contribute to sleep disturbances and, ultimately, to insomnia.

Debunking common myths and misconceptions about sleep is also fundamental in managing expectations and reducing sleep-related anxiety. One of the most prevalent myths is that everyone needs eight hours of sleep. Sleep requirements actually vary from person to person and can change throughout life. Understanding that sleep needs are individual can alleviate some of the stress related to achieving a specific number of sleep hours and allow you to focus more on the quality of sleep and how you feel during your waking hours.

In this chapter, we will delve deeper into the mechanisms of sleep, the different types of insomnia, and their broad impact on mental, physical, and social health. By breaking down these elements, we aim to arm you with knowledge and strategies to improve your sleep, moving beyond mere definitions to practical applications and lifestyle adjustments that can significantly enhance your sleep quality and, by extension, your life.

The Science of Sleep: What Happens When You Can't Sleep

Sleep is an intricate and vital process, and understanding its structure is crucial for grasping how disruptions can lead to insomnia. The sleep cycle consists of several stages, classified into two main types: REM (Rapid Eye Movement) and non-REM sleep, each playing a unique role in brain health and function. Non-REM sleep itself is divided into three stages. The first is the lightest stage of sleep, where you can be easily awakened; it acts as a doorway to deeper sleep. The second stage is where your body begins to truly relax, with slower brain waves, decreased body temperature, and slowed heart rate. The third stage of non-REM sleep is the deepest and most restorative stage. During this stage, tissues grow and repair, energy is restored, and hormones crucial for growth and development are released. Following these stages, REM sleep occurs approximately 90 minutes after falling asleep and cycles back every 90 minutes. This stage is associated with dreaming, memory consolidation, and emotional processing. It is characterized by increased brain activity, rapid eye movements, and muscle paralysis, which prevents you from acting out your dreams.

The body's circadian rhythm regulates the orchestration of these sleep stages and is often called the body's internal clock. External light cues influence this natural timer and dictate physical, mental, and behavioral changes over 24 hours. One of its most crucial roles is determining sleep patterns. It helps regulate the timing of when sleep occurs by controlling the release of melatonin, the hormone that promotes sleepiness. When this rhythm is disrupted by factors such as light pollution, irregular sleep schedules, or jet lag, it can lead to difficulty falling asleep, staying asleep, or experiencing restorative sleep, all hallmarks of insomnia.

The consequences of sleep loss extend far beyond feeling drowsy. Short-term impacts include impaired cognitive function, such as decreased concentration and reduced decision-making skills, and emotional effects, such as irritability and reduced stress tolerance. Long-term sleep deprivation can have more severe health implications, including an increased risk of chronic conditions such as cardiovascular disease, diabetes, and obesity. Furthermore, prolonged sleep disruption can lead to significant mood disorders like depression and anxiety, creating a vicious cycle where sleep quality and mental health continuously deteriorate each other.

Neurochemicals play pivotal roles in both the initiation and maintenance of sleep. Melatonin, often known as the 'sleep hormone,' is produced in response to darkness and signals the body to prepare for sleep. Its levels rise in the evening and stay elevated throughout the night, promoting consistent and restful sleep. Cortisol, the 'stress hormone,' typically counteracts melatonin and is involved in the wakefulness part of the circadian rhythm. Normally, cortisol levels increase in the early morning to promote wakefulness and alertness and decrease at night to allow melatonin to take over. However, when stress or irregular sleep patterns disrupt this balance, elevated nighttime cortisol levels can lead to wakefulness and fragmented sleep patterns, which are common complaints in those with insomnia.

Understanding these processes highlights why a regular sleep schedule and a conducive sleeping environment are crucial for quality rest. It also underscores the importance of addressing any underlying issues that may disrupt these delicate hormonal balances, such as stress or irregular lifestyle habits, to combat insomnia effectively. By aligning our sleep habits with our natural biological rhythms and ensuring our neurochemicals are balanced, we can foster better sleep health and reduce the likelihood of insomnia, paving the way for more energized and productive days.

Types of Insomnia and Identifying Your Pattern

Insomnia, often considered a general term for sleep trouble, actually encompasses a variety of conditions, each with its own characteristics and challenges. To effectively address and manage insomnia, it's crucial to understand its various forms and identify patterns in your sleep that signify specific types. Acute insomnia, a brief episode of difficulty sleeping, is usually triggered by life circumstances such as stress from an upcoming work event or sadness from a recent loss. This type of insomnia tends to resolve without treatment once the precipitating factor is removed. In contrast, chronic insomnia is defined by symptoms that occur at least three nights a week for more than three months. Chronic insomnia is more complex and often involves deeper biological or psychological issues.

Beyond these broad categories, insomnia also varies in its specificity. Situational insomnia occurs in specific contexts or environments that disrupt sleep—for instance, an uncomfortable hotel room during travel. Recurrent insomnia, on the other hand, involves repeated episodes of sleep disruption interspersed with periods of normal sleep, often triggered by recurring stressors or lifestyle patterns. Idiopathic insomnia, a lifelong sleep disorder, begins in childhood and progresses into adulthood without an identifiable cause. Understanding these distinctions is pivotal in crafting a targeted approach to improving sleep.

Identifying personal patterns of insomnia involves more than noting the hours of missed sleep. It requires meticulous attention to the conditions and habits surrounding your sleep environment and routines. One effective method is maintaining a sleep diary. By diligently recording details like bedtime, wake-up time, total sleep time, perceived sleep quality, and feelings upon waking, you can begin to recognize patterns and triggers that affect your sleep. This might include obvious factors like caffeine consumption close to bedtime or more subtle ones like emotional stressors. Environmental factors, such as noise levels or exposure to light, can also significantly disrupt sleep patterns and are important to document.

Secondary insomnia is another crucial concept to understand. It refers to sleep problems that occur as a symptom of another medical condition, such as anxiety, depression, arthritis, or heart disease. In such cases, while the sleep disorder itself needs to be addressed, effective management also involves treating the underlying health issue. For example, treating depression might also alleviate insomnia associated with it, as these conditions often feed into each other, creating a cycle of sleepless nights and gloomy days.

To illustrate, consider the case of a middle-aged professional who began experiencing sleep disturbances during a particularly stressful period at work. Initially, it seemed like a typical scenario of acute insomnia, where sleep would naturally improve as work stress diminished. However, the problem persisted over time, turning into a chronic condition. A deeper examination revealed underlying anxiety, not fully addressed by temporary stress management strategies. Treatment for anxiety alongside direct interventions for insomnia proved crucial in restoring healthier sleep patterns.

Another instance involves a woman in her late twenties who suffered from recurrent insomnia. She noticed that her sleep issues would spike during winter, a pattern that emerged over several years. This pattern was initially perplexing until she learned about Seasonal Affective Disorder (SAD), a type of depression related to changes in seasons, often triggering insomnia in its sufferers. Understanding the link between her mood fluctuations and sleep patterns allowed her to seek appropriate treatment for SAD, which in turn alleviated her sleep disturbances.

These examples underscore the importance of correctly identifying the type of insomnia and any underlying issues. Such insights guide more effective treatment strategies and empower individuals to make informed decisions about their health and well-being. As we continue to explore insomnia, remember that each scenario is unique, requiring personalized adjustments and interventions tailored to individual needs and conditions.

How Insomnia Affects Mental and Physical Health

Insomnia does not merely rob you of your sleep; it can profoundly impact both your mental and physical health, often creating a complex web of interrelated issues. It's crucial to understand the bidirectional relationship between insomnia and mental health disorders such as depression and anxiety. These relationships illustrate a cyclical dilemma where the presence of a mental health issue can lead to insomnia. Conversely, persistent insomnia may lead to the development or worsening of mental health conditions. For instance, anxiety about sleep itself can exacerbate insomnia, creating a distressing cycle that is difficult to break. Sleep deprivation has been shown to affect the brain's ability to regulate emotions. It can amplify feelings of sadness or anxiety, thus potentially triggering depression or escalating its severity if already present.

Chronic insomnia can also have significant repercussions on physical health. Prolonged sleep disruption can affect cardiovascular health, evidenced by increased risks of hypertension, heart disease, and stroke. These risks are compounded by the body's compromised ability to regulate stress hormones and blood pressure, both of which are closely tied to sleep quality. Furthermore, insomnia can influence metabolic processes, weight management, and the risk of type 2 diabetes. Sleep deprivation affects the body's ability to process glucose efficiently and regulate appetite, often leading to increased hunger and calorie intake, which can cause weight gain and heighten diabetes risk. The immune system is also less effective without adequate sleep. This reduction in immune function makes it harder to fight off infections and slows recovery from illness.

The cognitive impairments associated with sleep loss are both immediate and distressing. Memory retention, attention to detail, and decision-making capabilities are notably diminished when you sleep-deprived. This occurs because sleep is critical in memory consolidation and the neural connections supporting cognitive function and brain plasticity. Without enough rest, the brain struggles to encode new information and retrieve existing information. The lack of sleep also impairs judgment, leading to poor decision-making and increased risk-taking behavior, which can have serious personal and professional repercussions.

Beyond cognitive and physiological effects, insomnia significantly influences emotional and behavioral health. Chronic sleep deprivation can lead to mood swings, irritability, and decreased tolerance for stress, impacting social interactions and overall quality of life. The emotional regulation, which normally occurs during sleep, is disrupted, leading to heightened emotional reactivity. Individuals who have insomnia often report feeling more quick-tempered, prone to frustration, and generally more overwhelmed by daily stresses than they do when well-rested. This emotional volatility not only strains personal and professional relationships but can also exacerbate feelings of anxiety and depression, further entrenching the cycle of sleeplessness.

Understanding these far-reaching impacts of insomnia underscores the importance of addressing sleep issues not just for the sake of better rest but for maintaining overall health and well-being. As we continue to explore the complexities of insomnia, it becomes clear that its effects are not confined to the night alone; they extend into every aspect of life, shaping health, mood, cognitive abilities, and even social interactions. Each of these elements is deeply interwoven, suggesting that improvements in sleep can have far-reaching benefits beyond what might initially be imagined.

The Social and Economic Cost of Sleepless Nights

The ripple effects of insomnia extend far beyond the confines of the bedroom, permeating into various facets of social and economic life, often with significant consequences. At the workplace, the impact of sleep deprivation is both immediate and alarming. Individuals with insomnia will likely experience decreased productivity due to an inability to concentrate, slower reaction times, and a general decline in cognitive functions necessary for most tasks. The National Sleep Foundation reports that sleep deprivation is linked to a higher prevalence of errors and accidents at work. This affects individual performance and has broader organizational efficiency and safety implications. In industries where precision and alertness are critical, such as healthcare and transportation, the potential for catastrophic errors increases exponentially with sleep deprivation.

Furthermore, the effects of insomnia on work performance can lead to significant economic repercussions. Reduced productivity and increased errors contribute to financial losses for businesses. Additionally, the increased risk of workplace accidents leads to higher insurance costs and potential legal liabilities for companies. On a macroeconomic scale, studies suggest that sleep deprivation costs economies billions annually in lost productivity and healthcare expenditures. This economic burden is not just a corporate concern but a national one, impacting economic growth and healthcare systems worldwide.

Turning to personal relationships, insomnia's strain on social interactions is profound. Chronic sleep deprivation can lead to increased irritability and decreased patience, making interpersonal interactions more challenging. Sleep-deprived individuals often find it difficult to engage meaningfully with others, withdraw from social activities, or react too emotionally during normal conversations. This can strain relationships with family, friends, and colleagues, leading to social isolation and a decreased quality of life. Moreover, the lack of empathy and increased negativity often associated with poor sleep can erode relationships over time, leading to lasting impacts on one's social network and support systems.

The broader economic implications of insomnia are equally daunting. The healthcare costs associated with treating insomnia and its myriad complications are substantial. Beyond the direct costs of medical treatments and therapies for sleep disorders, there are significant expenditures related to managing the comorbidities associated with chronic insomnia, such as cardiovascular disease, obesity, diabetes, and mental health disorders. These conditions require long-term, costly interventions, which increase healthcare spending and economic strain on public and private insurers and individuals.

Additionally, the societal stigma surrounding sleeping disorders and mental health can profoundly affect individuals' willingness to seek help. There remains a pervasive attitude in many cultures that sleep issues are a sign of weakness or a minor problem that can be easily fixed. This stigma can prevent individuals from seeking professional help or even acknowledging their struggles, leading to a worsening of symptoms and a further increase in associated costs and health repercussions. The reluctance to discuss sleep problems openly also hampers public and organizational policies aimed at addressing this critical issue, perpetuating a cycle of silence and suffering.

These societal and economic challenges underscore the critical need for a broad-based approach to managing insomnia, including better public education, more robust workplace policies to support sleep health, and a reduction in the stigma associated with sleep disorders. We aim to mitigate these extensive costs and improve the quality of life for millions suffering from insomnia by acknowledging the importance of sleep and proactive strategies to promote and protect sleep health. As we continue to explore and address these issues, it becomes increasingly clear that the fight against insomnia is not just a personal health issue but a societal imperative.

Chapter Two

Psychological Triggers of Insomnia

Imagine lying in bed enveloped by darkness as the clock ticks past midnight. You're exhausted, yet your mind races with endless thoughts about tasks undone and challenges ahead. This scenario is all too familiar for many, where the quiet of the night becomes a stage for anxiety's performance, disrupting sleep and peace of mind. In this chapter, we delve into the intricate relationship between psychological states like stress and anxiety and their impact on sleep, uncovering the mechanisms behind these interactions and offering practical solutions to reclaim the night.

Stress and Anxiety: The Sleep Stealers

Stress and anxiety are notorious for their ability to disrupt sleep. They activate the body's fight or flight response, releasing hormones like adrenaline and cortisol that increase alertness and energy, mechanisms that are evolutionary designed to protect us from threats. However, when this response is triggered at night by worries or stress, it becomes a barrier to the peaceful slumber your body so desperately needs. The heightened state of alertness keeps the mind engaged in a whirlwind of activity that can make sleep seem like an impossible goal.

Symptoms of anxiety that typically invade the night include racing thoughts, where your mind continuously cycles through worries and fears, and excessive worrying about past events or future possibilities. Physically, you might experience heart palpitations, an accelerated heart rate that further signals your body to stay awake and alert. These symptoms are not only distressing but also conducive to a state of hyperarousal that is antithetical to the calm required for sleep.

Specific relaxation techniques can be immensely beneficial in counteracting anxiety-induced insomnia. Deep breathing exercises, for example, help mitigate the physiological symptoms of anxiety by slowing the heart rate and promoting relaxation. Techniques such as the 4-7-8 breathing method, where you breathe in for four seconds, hold the breath for seven seconds, and exhale slowly over eight seconds, can be particularly effective.

Mindfulness meditation is another powerful tool. It involves focusing your attention on the present moment and observing your thoughts and feelings without judgment. This practice can help break the cycle of anxiety by reducing the tendency to ruminate on worries, thus easing the mind into a state more conducive to sleep. Journaling before bed can also be therapeutic; it allows you to download your thoughts and concerns onto paper, which can help clear your mind and ease the anxiety that often builds up with the prospect of sleep.

Consider the case of Michael, a project manager in his late thirties, who found himself overtaken by anxiety at night, his mind buzzing with deadlines and deliverables. His sleep suffered terribly, leaving him tired and even more stressed during the day. By incorporating mindfulness meditation and journaling into his nightly routine, Michael was able to calm his mind and significantly improve his sleep. He noted that meditating helped him set aside his work-related worries at night, and journaling gave him a sense of closure from the day's stresses, preparing him for sleep.

Interactive Element: Journaling Prompt

To apply a similar strategy to Michael's, try this simple exercise: Each night, spend five minutes writing down the main worries on your mind. Next to each worry, write a brief note on whether it's something within your control or not. For those within your control, jot down a small step you might take the next day to address it. For those beyond your control, remind yourself that worrying will not change the outcome. This practice can help categorize your thoughts and reduce the burden they impose at night.

In exploring these dynamics and tools, we find that while stress and anxiety are formidable opponents of sleep, they are not insurmountable. With the proper techniques and a bit of practice, you can manage these nighttime disruptions and pave the way for more peaceful and restorative sleep.

Depression and Its Ties to Insomnia

Depression and insomnia often intertwine in a complex dance, each influencing and exacerbating the other in a cyclical relationship that can challenge the very core of well-being. When you are depressed, you may find that sleep, which should be a refuge, becomes elusive or unsatisfying. Conversely, the lack of restorative sleep can deepen and prolong depressive episodes, creating a cycle that feels impossible to break. Understanding this relationship is crucial for anyone seeking to manage these conditions effectively.

The interaction between depression and sleep disturbances manifests in various ways. One of the most common symptoms related to both conditions is early morning wakefulness, where you might find yourself waking up hours earlier than needed, unable to go back to sleep. This symptom can exacerbate the feelings of sadness and hopelessness that accompany depression, as the quiet, early hours may lead to negative ruminations with little distraction. Another symptom is hypersomnia, where you find yourself sleeping excessively yet not feeling rested. This excessive sleep can interfere with daily activities and responsibilities, increasing feelings of guilt and worthlessness, which are often associated with depression.

Addressing these intertwined issues often requires a multifaceted approach. Treating depression can lead to significant improvements in sleep quality and vice versa. Psychotherapy, particularly cognitive behavioral therapy (CBT), has been effective in treating both depression and insomnia. CBT focuses on identifying and changing negative thought patterns and behaviors contributing to both conditions. For instance, CBT for insomnia (CBT-I) helps modify thoughts and behaviors that prevent restful sleep, while CBT for depression targets patterns that exacerbate sadness and hopelessness.

Pharmacological treatments can also play a role, though they should be carefully considered under the guidance of a healthcare professional. Antidepressants can help alleviate the symptoms of depression, and some have properties that aid in improving sleep. However, it's important to note that some medications might have side effects affecting sleep, underscoring the need for a careful, personalized approach to pharmacotherapy.

Seeking professional help is a crucial step in effectively managing the interplay between depression and insomnia. It's important to consult with healthcare providers who understand the complexities of both conditions. They can offer a comprehensive evaluation and tailor treatment plans that address both mental health and sleep, providing a more holistic approach to recovery. If you find yourself consistently struggling with sleep and mood disturbances, it is advisable to reach out for professional help. Early intervention can prevent the conditions from becoming more entrenched and difficult to manage.

In practical terms, managing the relationship between depression and insomnia involves more than just treatment—it requires an understanding and adjustment of lifestyle habits and routines. Creating a bedtime routine that encourages relaxation, limiting exposure to screens before bed, and ensuring your sleep environment is conducive to rest can all help improve sleep quality. Simultaneously, engaging in regular physical activity, maintaining a healthy diet, and staying connected with supportive friends or family can help manage and alleviate symptoms of depression. By addressing both conditions simultaneously and with various tools, you stand a better chance of breaking the cycle and improving your sleep and mood significantly.

This holistic approach to managing depression and its impact on sleep is not just about treating symptoms but about fostering a lifestyle conducive to mental health and restorative sleep. By understanding the deep connections between how you feel and how you sleep, you can begin to make changes that will profoundly impact your overall quality of life, moving beyond the disruptions of depression and insomnia to a more balanced and fulfilling daily experience.

PTSD and Nightmares: Processing Trauma

Trauma doesn't quietly fade away when it enters a person's life. Instead, it can linger, invading nights with nightmares and disturbed sleep, making rest seem like an unattainable luxury. Individuals who have Post-Traumatic Stress Disorder (PTSD) often experience profound disruptions in their sleep patterns, a testament to the deep-seated impact of traumatic experiences. These disruptions can include a range of sleep disturbances from insomnia to nightmare disorder, where vivid, disturbing dreams frequently interrupt sleep, often leading to a fear of sleeping and a vicious cycle of sleep avoidance and anxiety.

The link between PTSD and sleep disturbances primarily centers around the persistent state of hyperarousal intrinsic to PTSD. This condition keeps the body's fight-or-flight response on high alert, leading to an increased heart rate, rapid breathing, and a flood of stress hormones—conditions fundamentally incompatible with the calm required for sleep. The brain, sensing danger, remains vigilant, disrupting the normal progression into deep, restorative sleep stages. Nightmares, a common symptom for those with PTSD, often replay elements of the trauma or create new scenarios with similar themes of danger and helplessness, further preventing restful sleep.

Addressing these complex sleep issues often requires a multifaceted therapeutic approach. Trauma-focused Cognitive Behavioral Therapy (CBT), a specialized branch of CBT, is designed to work through traumatic memories and change the distressing patterns of thought and behavior that result from traumatic experiences. This type of therapy helps to lessen the grip of trauma on an individual's life, which can, in turn, alleviate associated sleep disturbances.

Another impactful therapy is Eye Movement Desensitization and Reprocessing (EMDR), which has been particularly effective for those haunted by traumatic memories and nightmares. EMDR involves the rhythmic shifting of eye movements while recalling a traumatic event. This process can help the brain reprocess traumatic memories in a way that reduces their emotional impact, potentially decreasing the frequency and intensity of nightmares and improving overall sleep quality.

Imagery rehearsal therapy (IRT) is yet another approach specifically aimed at those plagued by nightmares. This technique involves changing the ending of the remembered nightmare while awake, rehearsing the new, non-threatening outcome in the mind. This practice can help modify the narrative of the nightmares, making them less frightening and disruptive. Over time, IRT can help reduce the occurrence of nightmares and improve sleep quality by decreasing nighttime anxiety and improving one's sense of control over their dreams.

For those coping with PTSD and related sleep disturbances, accessing professional guidance and support is crucial. Many resources are available, including PTSD support groups where individuals can share experiences and coping strategies in a supportive environment, enhancing feelings of understanding and community. Professional therapists specializing in PTSD can offer personalized therapy sessions, utilizing techniques like CBT, EMDR, or IRT tailored to individual needs. Additionally, online resources, like the National Center for PTSD [https://www.ptsd.va.gov/], provide extensive information and tools for managing PTSD-related sleep issues.

Navigating the interplay between trauma, PTSD, and sleep is undoubtedly challenging. Still, with the right therapeutic approaches and support systems, it is possible to improve sleep quality and find relief from the nocturnal grip of trauma. As we continue to explore these methods and their applications, the hope is that those affected by PTSD can find not only solace but also a path to better, more restorative sleep.

The Role of Chronic Stress in Chronic Insomnia

Chronic stress, a persistent state of tension and strain, can be precipitated by ongoing pressures from various facets of life, such as work demands, long-term health issues, or continuous relationship conflicts. Unlike acute stress, a brief and often intense response to a specific event, chronic stress lingers, embedding itself into your daily life so subtly that you might not notice its presence until it manifests through physical or emotional symptoms. This type of stress does not just fade away with the resolution of a situation; it is sustained over time, gradually undermining both mental and physical health and significantly disrupting sleep patterns.

The relationship between chronic stress and sleep is particularly insidious. Prolonged exposure to stress leads to an overproduction of cortisol, a hormone that is part of the body's fight-or-flight response. While cortisol is beneficial in short bursts and necessary for survival situations, its continuous presence in your system can wreak havoc, particularly on your sleep-wake cycle. Elevated cortisol levels at night keep your body in a state of hyperarousal, counteracting the natural decrease in cortisol that should occur as evening progresses. This hormonal imbalance not only makes it difficult to fall asleep but also to maintain deep sleep, leading to a night of restless tossing and turning. Over time, the lack of restorative sleep can exacerbate the stress, creating a destructive cycle where each condition perpetuates the other.

Addressing chronic stress and its impact on sleep requires a multi-faceted approach, emphasizing long-term strategies rather than quick fixes. One effective method is engaging in regular physical activity, which has been shown to decrease overall cortisol levels and improve mood by releasing endorphins, known as the body's natural painkillers and mood elevators. However, the timing of exercise is crucial; engaging in vigorous activities close to bedtime can have the opposite effect, increasing cortisol levels and delaying sleep. Therefore, scheduling morning or early afternoon workouts is generally best for improving nighttime sleep quality.

Equally important is the establishment of a consistent daily routine. The human body thrives on predictability, and setting a regular schedule for waking, eating, working, and sleeping can help regulate your internal clock, reducing the physiological impacts of stress. This routine should also include dedicated time for relaxation and unwinding before bed, which can involve reading, taking a warm bath, or engaging in relaxation exercises like yoga or meditation. These activities help transition your body into a state of readiness for sleep and provide a mental break from the day's stress, allowing you to approach bedtime with a calmer mind.

Moreover, implementing stress management programs can be tremendously beneficial. These programs often include techniques such as mindfulness meditation, cognitive behavioral therapy, and stress reduction workshops that teach you how to manage stressors more effectively and reduce overall anxiety. By learning to address and mitigate the sources of chronic stress, you can significantly lessen its impact on your sleep quality. Additionally, setting boundaries in both personal and professional life is essential to prevent stress from becoming overwhelming. This might involve learning to say no to additional responsibilities, delegating tasks when possible, or simply ensuring you have time set aside each day for self-care.

Incorporating these strategies into your life may not eliminate stress entirely, but it can diminish its intensity and frequency, thereby improving your ability to achieve and maintain restful sleep. By actively managing stress through lifestyle adjustments, therapeutic practices, and routine setting, you can create a healthier balance in your life, paving the way for better sleep and overall well-being.

Breaking the Cycle: Cognitive Techniques That Help

Cognitive Behavioral Therapy (CBT), a form of psychotherapy, has proven highly effective not just in managing mental health disorders but also in addressing the cognitive aspects of insomnia. This therapy focuses on identifying and changing dysfunctional thoughts and beliefs about sleep that often perpetuate sleep disturbances. For many, insomnia is fueled not just by external factors but also by a mental feedback loop where negative thoughts about sleep lead to anxiety and poor sleep habits, which in turn reinforce these negative thoughts.

One of the core components of CBT for insomnia is cognitive restructuring, a technique aimed at challenging and changing unhelpful beliefs about sleep. For instance, many individuals with insomnia often catastrophize the consequences of poor sleep, such as believing that if they don't get eight hours of sleep, they will not be able to function the next day. This belief puts undue pressure on the act of sleeping, which, ironically, makes sleep more elusive. Cognitive restructuring involves identifying such distorted thinking patterns and challenging their validity. It encourages questioning the evidence for such beliefs, the actual consequences of poor sleep, and the possibility of other outcomes. For example, by reflecting on past experiences, you might realize that while you feel tired after a poor night's sleep, you can still function effectively, thus disproving the belief that poor sleep completely incapacitates you.

Incorporating behavior modification strategies is another crucial aspect of CBT that can significantly improve sleep. Techniques such as stimulus control and sleep restriction are commonly used. Stimulus control involves using the bed only for sleep and sex, thereby strengthening the association between the bed and sleep. If unable to sleep, the recommendation is to leave the bed and return only when sleepy. This prevents the bed from becoming a battleground of tossing and turning, which can worsen insomnia. On the other hand, sleep restriction limits the amount of time spent in bed to only the actual sleep time, which can help consolidate sleep and increase sleep efficiency. If you typically spend eight hours in bed but only sleep for five, sleep restriction would involve initially limiting the time in bed to five hours and gradually increasing it as sleep efficiency improves.

To engage you actively in these techniques, CBT often involves guided exercises or worksheets that you can incorporate into your daily routine. For instance, a sleep diary can be a practical tool, helping you track sleep patterns and identify behaviors or thoughts that might be detrimental to sleep. This proactive engagement enhances your understanding of your sleep patterns and empowers you to make informed adjustments to improve sleep quality.

By integrating these cognitive and behavioral strategies, CBT provides a robust framework for tackling insomnia. It shifts the focus from external sleep aids to internal cognitive processes, offering a more sustainable solution to sleep issues. Moreover, the skills learned through CBT, such as anxiety management and cognitive restructuring, can also benefit other areas of life, providing a comprehensive approach to wellness.

As we wrap up this exploration of how cognitive techniques can help break the cycle of insomnia, we see the mind's power in disturbing and restoring sleep. Understanding and modifying our thoughts and behaviors around sleep can transform how we approach the night—from a time of potential stress and frustration to rest and renewal. These techniques not only enhance our ability to sleep but also improve our overall mental resilience, equipping us to handle whatever challenges life may throw our way.

In the next chapter, we will delve into the physiological strategies for combatting insomnia, exploring how adjustments to diet, exercise, and other lifestyle factors can further enhance our sleep quality and overall health. This holistic approach, combining cognitive techniques with physical health strategies, offers the most effective path to conquering insomnia and reclaiming the restorative power of sleep.

Chapter Three

Lifestyle and Environmental Adjustments

Imagine entering a room where each element has been thoughtfully placed to invite calmness and tranquility—a sanctuary where the day's chaos dissolves at the threshold. This isn't just a daydream for those searching for spa-like retreats; it's a practical blueprint for transforming your bedroom into a sleep sanctuary. In the quest to conquer insomnia, the environment where you sleep plays a pivotal role, not just in the hours spent in bed but in setting the stage for your entire night's rest. This chapter guides you through optimizing your bedroom to foster conditions that enhance sleep quality, turning it into a haven of rest.

Creating Your Sleep Sanctuary: Optimizing Your Bedroom

Prioritize Minimalism and Organization

A cluttered room reflects a cluttered mind, and both are detrimental to achieving peaceful slumber. The first step in creating your sleep sanctuary is to embrace minimalism in your bedroom setup. This doesn't mean your space should feel stark or devoid of personality, but each element in the room should serve a purpose and contribute to an overarching sense of calm. Start by decluttering—remove items unrelated to sleep or relaxation, such as work materials, exercise equipment, or any clutter that could distract from the room's primary purpose: rest. The less clutter, the more your mind can relax and prepare for sleep. An organized and tidy bedroom minimizes distractions and decreases the cognitive load that can keep you alert when you should be winding down.

Choose the Right Bedding and Mattress

Your bed should be a welcoming embrace, ready to comfort you after a long day. The choice of mattress, pillows, and bed linens plays a crucial role as they directly affect your comfort and, consequently, your sleep quality. A mattress should properly support your body's natural posture, maintain the spine's natural curve, and support your head, shoulders, hips, and feet. The firmness of the mattress should be guided by personal preference and specific bodily needs. For instance, some may require a firmer mattress to alleviate back pain, while others might prefer something softer. Pillows should also be chosen based on sleeping positions; for example, side sleepers generally need thicker pillows to keep their neck aligned with the rest of their spine, whereas stomach sleepers might benefit from softer, thinner pillows.

Similarly, the textures and fabrics of your bed linens can enhance sleep. Natural fibers like cotton or bamboo are breathable and help regulate body temperature, making them an excellent choice for sheets and comforters. These materials can help prevent overheating during the night, a common complaint that can disrupt sleep. Additionally, choosing the right bedding involves considering hypoallergenic options if you suffer from allergies. Dust mites, pet dander, and other allergens can accumulate in bedding and interrupt sleep through respiratory distress or skin irritation, making hypoallergenic materials a wise choice for sensitive individuals.

Consider the Color and Decor

The color palette of your bedroom can significantly influence your mood and relaxation levels. Colors can evoke emotions; for instance, blues and greens are often associated with calmness and serenity, making them ideal choices for a sleep environment. These colors tend to lower blood pressure and heart rate, which are conducive to relaxation and sleep. On the other hand, bright colors like reds and oranges stimulate the mind and energy levels, which is counterproductive in a sleep setting.

When decorating, aim for simplicity and personal comfort. Artwork can be soothing but should not be emotionally charged or stimulating. The decor should reflect tranquility and comfort, creating a personalized and restful environment. Soft, ambient lighting can also enhance the peacefulness of the room; consider installing dimmers or using lamps with warm-toned bulbs to help signal to your body that it's time to wind down. The setup of your room should invite relaxation, making it clear that this space is dedicated to rest.

Optimize Bedroom Layout for Sleep

The furniture arrangement and your bed's orientation can also impact your sleep quality. Your bed should be positioned in a way that feels secure and protected. According to the principles of Feng Shui, the bed should be in a "command position," meaning it faces the door but is not directly in line with it. This placement provides a sense of safety and control, reducing anxiety and promoting relaxation. Additionally, ensure your bed has a clear path on both sides, offering convenience and a balance of energy in the room.

Minimizing external noise and light is also crucial. If external light or sounds are an issue, consider using heavy curtains, blackout shades, or double-pane windows. These adjustments can shield you from disruptions that might otherwise disturb your sleep, such as street lights or traffic noise. The goal is to control the environment as much as possible to suit your specific needs, making your bedroom a true sanctuary that supports deep, restorative sleep.

Every element should contribute to a greater sense of peace and relaxation when transforming your bedroom into a sleep sanctuary. From the color of the walls to the feel of your sheets, each choice is a step towards better sleep. This chapter sets the foundation for this transformation, guiding you through choices, large and small, that can make significant differences in your sleep quality. As we continue to explore the adjustments you can make in your living environment, remember that the goal is not just to sleep but to sleep well, embracing each night with the peace and comfort you deserve.

The Impact of Light: Natural and Artificial Influences

Light is fundamental in regulating our sleep patterns, significantly influencing our internal biological clock or circadian rhythm. This internal clock manages the timing of various physiological processes, including the sleep-wake cycle. It is finely tuned to the natural light-dark cycle of our environment, which historically has been dictated by the sun's rising and setting. Exposure to light significantly impacts melatonin production, often referred to as the 'sleep hormone,' which is secreted by the pineal gland in the brain primarily in response to darkness. Melatonin levels rise in the evening, promoting sleepiness, and fall in the morning, helping us wake up. This natural ebb and flow of melatonin are crucial for maintaining a healthy sleep cycle.

However, in our modern environment, we're often exposed to various sources of artificial light, which can disrupt this natural rhythm. Blue light, which is emitted at a high level by electronic devices such as smartphones, tablets, and computers, as well as energy-efficient LED lighting, is particularly disruptive. It has a short wavelength that affects melatonin levels more than any other wavelength. Exposure to blue light in the hours before bedtime can trick the brain into thinking it's still daytime, which reduces melatonin production and makes it harder to fall asleep.

To mitigate the impact of blue light on sleep, consider adopting specific strategies to manage your exposure. Using blue light filters on your devices, often built into many modern smartphones and computers, can help reduce blue light emissions. Alternatively, wearing glasses that block blue light can be an effective method, especially if you need to use these devices close to bedtime. Moreover, establishing a no-electronics rule in the hour leading up to sleep can further protect your natural sleep cycle. Instead of scrolling through social media or sending late-night emails, you can read a book, prepare for the next day, or engage in a relaxing hobby, which can help signal your body that it's time to wind down.

Beyond managing exposure to blue light, harnessing the power of natural light can enhance your sleep quality. Our bodies evolved to respond to the patterns of the sun, and aligning our sleep schedule more closely with natural light can help reinforce our circadian rhythms. Exposure to natural light, especially in the morning, can help reset our internal clocks daily. It signals the body that it's time to wake up and start the day. To incorporate more natural light into your routine, spend time outside in natural sunlight for at least 30 minutes each morning. If direct sunlight is scarce, especially during winter, a bright light therapy device can be a helpful substitute, simulating the sunrise to help your body wake up naturally.

In the evenings, the type of artificial lighting in your home can also help prepare your body for sleep. Opt for lamps with dimmable features and warm-toned bulbs that mimic the natural light of the sunset, which doesn't interfere with melatonin production as blue-toned lighting can. These lighting choices can create a cozy, relaxing atmosphere conducive to winding down. Consider setting your lights on timers to gradually decrease the amount of light in your environment as bedtime approaches, mimicking the natural transition from daylight to evening.

You can significantly enhance your sleep quality by understanding light's profound impact on your sleep and implementing strategies to optimize natural and artificial light exposure. Adjusting how and when you interact with various light sources throughout the day can help maintain your circadian rhythm, making it easier to fall asleep and wake up feeling refreshed. This adjustment to your light exposure is just one of the many ways you can fine-tune your environment and habits for better sleep, demonstrating how intertwined our biological systems are with the natural world.

Soundscapes for Sleep: Using Audio to Enhance Sleep Quality

The gentle hum of a distant fan, the rhythmic pattering of rain against the window, or the soothing symphony of forest sounds—audio environments can profoundly influence our ability to drift off into a peaceful slumber. In our quest to create optimal sleep conditions, considering the auditory landscape of our sleeping environment is as crucial as the physical setup. Introducing white noise and sound machines can be a game changer for many, particularly for those whose sleep is easily disrupted by irregular or jarring background noises.

White noise machines generate a consistent, ambient sound that spans a wide range of frequencies, effectively masking other sounds that might wake you from sleep. This could include traffic noise, the sudden bark of a dog, or even the intermittent sounds of a house settling. The consistent nature of white noise creates a buffer of sound that helps maintain a serene environment conducive to sustained sleep. For individuals living in busy urban environments or noisy neighborhoods, a white noise machine can be essential in their sleep toolkit. White noise is often likened to a soft hissing or static, which might seem counterintuitive as a sleep aid. Still, its uniformity is key—not the noise itself but the consistency and predictability that helps calm the mind and mask disruptive sounds.

Moving beyond white noise, the natural world offers a plethora of sounds that have been shown to aid relaxation and sleep. Nature sounds, such as rainfall, ocean waves, rustling leaves, or a flowing river, are naturally rhythmic and soothing. These sounds not only help reduce stress but also enhance the quality of sleep by promoting relaxation. These repetitive and predictable sounds can signal to the brain that it's time to wind down, preparing the body for sleep. Calming music, particularly compositions with a slow tempo and soft melodies, can also have a similar effect. The key is the tempo, typically around 60 beats per minute, which can help slow the heart rate and induce relaxation more profoundly than many other types of music.

Setting Up a Sleep-Friendly Audio Environment

Placing speakers or sound machines in your bedroom should be strategic to create an effective auditory environment for sleep. Ideally, the sound source should be a manageable distance from the bed to avoid overwhelming the ears or making it difficult to fall asleep. Instead, placing the device at a distance that allows the sound to fill the room gently can create an immersive soundscape that envelops you in soothing audio. Volume control is crucial; the sound should be loud enough to mask disruptive noises but not so loud that it becomes a disturbance. A moderate volume level that comfortably blends into the background is optimal.

When setting up your sleep-friendly audio environment, consider using a sound machine that offers a variety of sound options so you can choose the one that best suits your preferences. Many modern devices offer customizable settings, including volume adjustment, sound selection, and even timers that can turn the device off once you fall asleep. This feature is handy as it conserves energy and prevents changes in the audio environment from waking you later at night.

App and Device Recommendations

Several apps and devices can help create the perfect sleep soundscape for those looking to enhance their sleep through audio. Apps like "Calm" and "Noisli" offer a wide range of natural and ambient sounds, from thunderstorms and ocean waves to white noise and city ambiance. These apps often include features that allow you to mix sounds to your liking, adjust volumes, and set timers, making them highly versatile options for personalizing your sleep experience.

Sound machines such as the LectroFan Classic offer a variety of white noise, and fan sounds with precise volume control, making it easy to find the perfect setting for your needs. For a more high-tech solution, the Bose Sleepbuds II combines noise-masking technology and relaxing audio tracks in a comfortable earbud design that won't disturb your sleep even if you roll over or change positions at night.

In selecting apps and devices, look for options that offer a range of sounds. Experiment with different audio landscapes to discover what works best for you. Consider ease of use, especially if you'll be operating the device in a low-light environment, and check for any features that enhance usability, like automatic shut-offs or programmable settings.

Temperature and Comfort: Setting the Stage for Restful Sleep

Navigating the delicate balance of bedroom temperature can significantly enhance your sleep quality. Research consistently suggests that the ideal temperature for optimal sleep is around 65 degrees Fahrenheit (18 degrees Celsius), though this can vary slightly based on individual preferences. Cooler temperatures are generally conducive to better sleep because they help lower the body's core temperature, a necessary step for initiating sleep. As your body prepares for sleep, its internal temperature naturally drops, signaling to your brain that it's time to wind down. An environment that mirrors this natural cooling can facilitate this transition, making falling and staying asleep easier. Conversely, an environment that's too warm can hinder this process, leading to restless sleep and frequent awakenings.

To maintain this ideal sleeping climate, especially in seasons when the outside temperatures can drastically differ from your sleep-ideal setting, there are several strategies you can employ. Using a programmable thermostat can be particularly effective as it allows you to automate the temperature settings, ensuring your bedroom is always at your ideal temperature when it's time to sleep. Portable fans or air conditioners can be invaluable for those without the option of adjusting their home's thermostat. Positioning a fan strategically in your bedroom can help circulate air and maintain a cool environment. During colder months, consider layering blankets that can easily be removed if you get too warm rather than cranking up the heat. This way, you can adjust your bedding to maintain comfort without overheating.

The choice of bedding also plays a crucial role in temperature regulation throughout the night. Materials that wick moisture and allow your skin to breathe are pivotal in maintaining a comfortable sleep temperature. Moisture-wicking sheets, made from materials like bamboo, cotton, or specialized synthetic blends, draw sweat away from the body, helping to keep you dry and cool. Similarly, breathable comforters or duvets filled with natural fibers like wool or down can provide insulation while allowing air circulation, helping to regulate body temperature throughout the night. These bedding choices help maintain the ideal sleep temperature and enhance overall sleep comfort, contributing to a deeper and more restful night's sleep.

Temperature-related sleep disturbances, such as night sweats or chills, can be particularly challenging. For those who experience night sweats, moisture-wicking and breathable bedding are essential. Additionally, wearing light, breathable sleepwear can prevent overheating and reduce sweat production. Consider a cooling mattress pad or pillow, which can help draw heat away from the body for an extra cooling effect. Layering bedding can provide customized warmth for those who tend to sleep cold. Consider using flannel sheets or a down comforter, which offer warmth without excessive weight. Electric blankets or heated mattress pads with adjustable settings can also provide warmth as needed without overheating the bed.

Innovations in sleep technology have led to the development of wearable tech designed to regulate body temperature. Thermal sleepwear and temperature-regulating sleep trackers can adjust your microclimate by absorbing, storing, and releasing body heat as needed. These technologies can benefit those with significant temperature-related sleep issues, providing a personalized solution to enhance sleep quality.

By understanding and optimizing the temperature and comfort of your sleep environment, you can create conditions that support your body's natural sleep processes. Adjusting the thermostat, selecting appropriate bedding, or utilizing temperature-regulating technologies can help you achieve a deeper, more restorative sleep. As we continue exploring how environmental factors influence sleep, remember that small changes in your sleep setting can significantly improve your overall sleep experience. These adjustments, tailored to your needs and preferences, can transform your bedroom into the ideal sleep sanctuary, fostering nights of quality rest.

Detox Your Evening Routine: Habits to Avoid Before Bed

Establishing a calming evening routine plays a pivotal role in easing the transition from the day's hustle to the peaceful repose of night. This process begins with a mindful approach to what we consume and engage with in the hours leading up to bedtime.

For starters, it is crucial to identify and avoid stimulants that can disrupt sleep. Substances like caffeine and nicotine are notorious for their stimulating effects on the central nervous system, which can delay the timing of sleep and reduce the total nightly sleep time. Caffeine found not only in coffee but also in tea, chocolate, some soft drinks, and certain medications can remain elevated in your blood for 6-8 hours. Therefore, coffee in the late afternoon can still linger in your system at bedtime. Similarly, nicotine, a stimulant found in cigarettes, can make it significantly harder to fall asleep. It's advisable to cut off caffeine consumption by the early afternoon and to avoid nicotine altogether, especially near bedtime, to help your body prepare for sleep naturally.

Equally disruptive can be consuming large or heavy meals late in the evening. Eating big or rich foods can lead to discomfort from indigestion, which can significantly impact your sleep quality. It's recommended to have your last large meal at least 2-3 hours before you plan to sleep. However, if you find yourself hungry close to bedtime, opt for a light snack, preferably rich in complex carbohydrates or a small amount of protein, which can aid in promoting sleep. Foods like a banana with peanut butter or a small bowl of whole-grain cereal with milk can be good choices that satisfy hunger without overtaxing your digestive system.

Another aspect to consider is the activities you engage in during the evening. Physically and psychologically stimulating activities, such as intense exercise or work-related tasks, can increase alertness and make it difficult to wind down. While regular exercise is highly beneficial for sleep and overall health, it should ideally be done earlier in the day. Instead, focus on more relaxing activities as bedtime approaches. This might include reading a book, listening to soft music, or practicing relaxation exercises such as gentle yoga or deep breathing. These activities help reduce stress and signal to your body that it's time to slow down and prepare for sleep.

Promote a Pre-Sleep Wind-Down Ritual

Creating a pre-sleep wind-down ritual is essential in preparing your mind and body for a good night's rest. This ritual can be personalized but should include activities that help you detach from the day's stresses and cue your body for sleep. For instance, developing the habit of meditating each night before bed can be particularly effective. Meditation helps to clear your mind of the day's clutter and ease stress, enhancing your ability to fall asleep and improving sleep quality throughout the night.

Similarly, incorporating gentle stretching into your evening routine can help relax your muscles and reduce physical tension, often accumulating throughout the day. These stretches need not be vigorous or strenuous but should be simple enough to perform at home, focusing on alleviating tension in areas like the neck, shoulders, and back.

Establishing such a routine eases the transition into sleep and enhances sleep quality. By consistently engaging in these relaxing activities before bed, you create an influential association in your mind between them and sleep, making it easier to fall asleep quickly and sleep more deeply over time.

As we conclude this chapter on optimizing your lifestyle and environment for better sleep, remember that these adjustments aim to create conditions that support your body's natural sleep processes. Whether it's through managing light exposure, optimizing your bedroom setup, or detoxing your evening routine, each strategy is geared towards enhancing the quality of your sleep. By making these changes, you not only improve your sleep but also your overall health and well-being.

The next chapter will explore psychological strategies to enhance sleep quality. We will address issues beyond the physical environment, including the cognitive and emotional realms that play critical roles in sleep health. Together, these strategies form a comprehensive approach to overcoming insomnia and achieving restful, restorative sleep.

Chapter Four

Diet, Exercise, and Sleep

As night descends and the world quiets, the quest for sleep begins—a quest that, for many, is fraught with challenges. What if the secret to unlocking restful sleep lies not in the silence of the night but in the choices made at the dinner table? In this chapter, we explore the profound impact of diet on sleep, delving into how the foods you eat can either invite restful slumber or summon the specters of sleeplessness.

Foods That Fight Insomnia: What to Eat and Avoid

Sleep-Promoting Foods

Imagine your body as a complex machine, where each component works harmoniously to transition you into a state of rest. Certain nutrients act as the cogs in this machine, facilitating the produc-

THE INSOMNIA BREAKTHROUGH: 41

tion of hormones crucial for sleep. Tryptophan, an amino acid found in turkey, is a star player in this process. It serves as a precursor to serotonin, a neurotransmitter that calms the mind, and as a critical building block for melatonin, the hormone directly involved in regulating sleep cycles. Almonds and other nuts offer a double benefit: rich in both tryptophan and magnesium, which has been shown to help reduce the occurrence of insomnia, particularly in older adults. Magnesium supports deep, restorative sleep by maintaining healthy levels of GABA, a neurotransmitter that promotes sleep.

Dairy products, often associated with the age-old advice of drinking a warm glass of milk before bed, also contain tryptophan and calcium. Calcium helps the brain use the tryptophan to manufacture melatonin. It's not just an old wives' tale; it's a science-backed strategy for better sleep. Incorporating these elements into your diet can enhance your body's ability to transition into sleep. For instance, a light snack of yogurt and a few almonds before bed can provide the right mix of tryptophan and magnesium to help usher in a peaceful night's sleep.

Foods to Avoid

Conversely, certain foods and beverages act more like sand in the gears of your sleep machine, disrupting the smooth transition into rest. Caffeine, a stimulant in coffee, tea, chocolate, and many sodas, is among the most common culprits. Its ability to ward off sleepiness is well-known, but you may need to realize that its effects can linger for several hours, making it a risky choice after mid-afternoon. Similarly, foods high in sugars and simple carbohydrates can trigger wakefulness at night by causing spikes in blood sugar levels, leading to a burst of energy at the wrong time. Heavy or rich foods, spicy dishes, and citrus fruits can cause discomfort, such as indigestion or acid reflux, mainly if consumed close to bedtime, making it hard to fall or stay asleep.

A Balanced Diet for Better Sleep

The key to diet's role in promoting good sleep lies in balance and timing. A well-rounded diet rich in vegetables, fruits, whole grains, lean proteins, and healthy fats supports overall health and regulates sleep patterns. These foods provide diverse nutrients necessary for synthesizing sleep-promoting hormones and maintaining a stable energy level throughout the day, which can help prepare the body for a restful night.

Meal Examples to Promote Good Sleep

To harness the power of diet in your quest for better sleep, consider meals that are easy on the stomach and rich in nutrients. A dinner of grilled salmon (rich in omega-3 fatty acids that may increase serotonin production), a side of jasmine rice, and steamed asparagus (both of which contain a modest amount of tryptophan) can set the stage for restful sleep. Alternatively, a light evening meal might include a turkey and avocado wrap with a side of cottage cheese, rounded off with a small banana. This combination offers a balance of tryptophan, magnesium, and calcium, all wrapped up in a satisfying yet not overly heavy meal.

Interactive Element: Journaling Your Diet and Sleep Patterns

To truly understand the impact of diet on your sleep, consider keeping a food and sleep journal. Track what you eat, particularly in the evening, and note the quality and duration of your sleep each night. This record can help you identify patterns and pinpoint which foods seem to disrupt your sleep and which seem to promote it. Over time, this journal can become a powerful tool for customizing your diet to enhance your sleep quality.

Understanding and adjusting what you eat can significantly influence how well you sleep. The relationship between diet and sleep is intricate and varies from person to person. Still, with careful attention and some experimentation, you can discover the dietary choices that best support your nighttime rest. As we continue to explore the connections between lifestyle choices and sleep, remember that each step you take towards balancing your diet is also a step towards reclaiming the restorative sleep you deserve.

Hydration and Sleep: Connecting Fluid Intake and Sleep Quality

Understanding the balance of fluid intake and its timing can play a pivotal role in enhancing sleep quality. It's a lesser-known fact that dehydration can significantly disrupt your sleep. Even mild dehydration can affect your sleep by triggering symptoms such as leg cramps, a common nocturnal annoyance that can jolt you awake from the most profound slumber. Additionally, dehydration often leads to a dry mouth or throat, which causes discomfort and can exacerbate snoring, further interrupting sleep. These disturbances underscore the importance of maintaining proper hydration to support uninterrupted sleep.

Maintaining optimal hydration involves more than just drinking plenty of fluids; it requires timing your intake to ensure it supports your sleep rather than detracts from it. During the day, aim to consume the majority of your fluids earlier on, tapering as the evening progresses. This approach helps to prevent the disruptive night-time trips to the bathroom that can fracture a night's sleep. Try to complete your fluid intake a few hours before bedtime. However, it's important to personalize this based on your body's signals and the specific needs that might vary from one person to another. For example, if you wake up at night feeling thirsty, a small glass of water might be necessary closer to bedtime. Listen to your body's cues to find a balance that suits your hydration needs without compromising your sleep.

In terms of what to drink before bed, certain beverages can be particularly beneficial for promoting sleep. Herbal teas, such as chamomile, valerian root, or lavender, are excellent choices. These teas contain compounds with natural sedative effects that can enhance sleep quality. They are hydrating and soothing, making them a perfect beverage for your nighttime routine. However, it's crucial to avoid drinks high in sugars or caffeine, such as certain sodas or black teas, close to bedtime. These can stimulate the nervous system and counteract the relaxation needed for sleep.

Hydration and Electrolytes: A Balancing Act

The role of electrolytes, such as potassium, magnesium, and calcium, in muscle function and hydration balance is well-documented, but their impact on sleep is equally significant. Electrolytes help regulate nerve function and muscle contractions — vital for quality rest. An imbalance in electrolytes can lead to sleep disturbances, including insomnia and frequent awakenings. For instance, low levels of magnesium are often associated with higher levels of stress and anxiety, which can make it harder to fall asleep. Similarly, insufficient potassium can lead to difficulty staying asleep due to its role in muscle health and relaxation.

Incorporating electrolyte-rich foods into your diet can be beneficial to ensure a proper balance of these crucial nutrients. Bananas are a great source of potassium, which assists in muscle relaxation and can help prevent disruptive leg cramps during the night. Spinach, rich in magnesium, supports muscle and nerve function and plays a role in melatonin synthesis, enhancing sleep quality. Including these foods in your dinner or as an evening snack can contribute to a better night's sleep by ensuring your electrolyte levels are balanced.

Staying adequately hydrated and maintaining electrolyte balance is vital for physical health and intricately linked to sleep quality. By managing your fluid intake thoughtfully throughout the day and choosing beverages and foods that support sleep, you can minimize sleep disruptions and enhance your overall sleep experience. This proactive approach to hydration and nutrition underscores the interconnectedness of your diet and sleep, providing another tool to combat insomnia and improve your nightly rest.

Timing Your Meals: How Eating Times Affect Sleep

In the balance of our daily rhythms, where our body's internal clocks meticulously orchestrate each step and turn, the timing of our meals plays a critical role in our digestion and sleep quality. Our digestive processes are intertwined with our circadian rhythms, the natural cycles that regulate various physiological processes, including sleep. Eating times, especially late in the evening, can significantly impact these rhythms, affecting sleep quality.

The circadian rhythm of digestion implies that our digestive system is more active during certain parts of the day, aligning with energy expenditure and metabolic needs. Our body begins to wind down as evening approaches, preparing for a restful night. The metabolic rate slows, and the body prepares for overnight fasting. Eating late at night can disrupt this natural progression, leading to indigestion or discomfort, keeping you awake, or disturbing your sleep. Furthermore, late meals can cause fluctuations in blood sugar levels, disrupt sleep, and affect your energy levels and mood the following day.

Therefore, the ideal timing for dinner is crucial for promoting good sleep. Finishing eating at least three to four hours before bedtime is generally recommended. This window allows enough time for your body to digest the meal and for your stomach to empty, reducing the likelihood of discomfort that might disturb your sleep. For instance, if you plan to sleep at 10 PM, aim to have dinner by 6 PM. This timing helps ensure that the digestive process aligns with your body's natural preparations for sleep, facilitating a smoother transition into rest.

Late-night snacking is another habit that can interfere with your sleep. While it's common to crave a snack after dinner, especially if there's a long gap between dinner and bedtime, the snack choice is crucial. High-fat, sugary, or large portions can rev up your metabolism, disrupting sleep. Instead, choosing small, nutritious snacks easy on the stomach can satisfy your hunger without impairing your sleep. For example, a small bowl of whole-grain cereal with milk, a banana, or a handful of nuts provides a good mix of complex carbohydrates and protein to produce sleep-inducing hormones.

Sample Daily Eating Schedule for Optimal Digestion and Sleep

To give you a clearer picture of how to align your eating habits with your sleep schedule, here's a sample daily eating schedule:

- **7:00 AM** - Breakfast: Eat a balanced breakfast with protein, healthy fats, and carbohydrates. For example, oatmeal with sliced almonds and berries paired with a cup of Greek yogurt.

- **Noon** - Lunch: A hearty lunch with lean protein, vegetables, and whole grains will sustain your energy levels throughout the afternoon. A grilled chicken salad with various vegetables and a vinaigrette dressing is a great option.

- **3:00 PM**—Snack: A small snack can help maintain your energy levels if you are hungry mid-afternoon. An apple with a handful of walnuts is an excellent choice.

- **6:00 PM**—Dinner: Aim to have your dinner early in the evening. Grilled salmon with quinoa and steamed broccoli provide a nutritious, light meal that's easy on the stomach.

- **8:00 PM**—Light Snack (optional): If you feel hungry before bed, a small, light snack can be acceptable. A warm glass of milk or a small banana can be soothing and help signal your body that it's time to wind down.

Following a schedule like this can help regulate your body's internal clock, improve digestion, and enhance your overall sleep quality. Consistency is key in maintaining circadian rhythms, so stick to similar eating times daily. This routine supports your body's natural processes and reinforces the daily rhythms that promote healthful sleep, allowing you to wake up refreshed and ready to tackle the day ahead.

Exercise for Sleep: Types and Timing

The gentle rhythm of your footsteps on the pavement as the evening sun dips below the horizon or the serene flow of a yoga sequence in the quiet of your living room—such activities are not just good for your physical health. Still, they are also crucial for your sleep. Regular physical activity significantly enhances the quality and duration of your sleep, particularly the proportion of restorative REM sleep. This deeper phase of sleep, characterized by rapid eye movement, is essential for cognitive functions such as memory consolidation and mood regulation. Regular exercise helps to increase the duration of REM phases throughout the night, allowing for a more restful and productive sleep cycle.

Exercise's ability to improve sleep is multifaceted. Physically, it helps expend energy, leading to a more pronounced feeling of tiredness at bedtime, naturally encouraging sleep onset. Moreover, exercise is a powerful stress reliever. It helps to reduce levels of the body's stress hormones, such as adrenaline and cortisol, which can interfere with sleep. During exercise, the release of endorphins, the body's natural painkillers and mood elevators, also plays a crucial role. These biochemicals help to foster a sense of well-being and relaxation, making it easier to wind down when it's time to sleep.

When considering the best types of exercise for promoting sleep, it's important to focus on activities that you enjoy and can perform consistently. Yoga, for example, is highly beneficial for sleep. Its combination of physical postures, controlled breathing, and meditation provides a holistic workout that reduces stress and anxiety, which are common culprits behind sleep disturbances. Light aerobic activities, such as walking or cycling, are also excellent. They help to raise your heart rate sufficiently to yield health benefits but are gentle enough not to interfere with nighttime relaxation.

Timing your exercise can be as important as the activity you choose. While vigorous exercise benefits your overall health, engaging in high-intensity workouts close to bedtime can be counterproductive. These activities stimulate the body, increasing heart rate and core body temperature, making it difficult to fall asleep. To promote evening relaxation, schedule vigorous workouts for earlier in the day. If you prefer to exercise in the evening, opt for more relaxing activities like gentle yoga or a leisurely walk. These exercises help to calm the mind and prepare the body for sleep, aligning with your natural circadian rhythms.

Relaxation Exercises Before Bedtime

To further enhance your pre-sleep routine, incorporating specific relaxation exercises can transition your body into restfulness, preparing you for a deep sleep. Gentle stretching or yoga can be particularly effective. These activities help relieve physical tension and calm the mind, easing the transition from wakefulness to sleep.

For example, consider incorporating poses such as the "legs-up-the-wall" pose, where you lie on your back with your legs extended vertically against a wall. This pose helps to relax the nervous system, lower blood pressure, and reduce heart rate, all of which are conducive to initiating sleep. Another helpful exercise is the seated forward bend, where you sit with your legs extended forward and gently lean your torso towards your thighs. This stretch can help alleviate stress and quiet your mind, making it easier to slip into sleep.

Integrating these exercises into your nightly routine signals your body that it's time to wind down and rest. Over time, this routine not only improves the quality of your sleep but also enhances your overall health, proving that a little movement—timed and chosen correctly—can pave the way to better nights and brighter mornings.

Supplements for Sleep: Melatonin and Beyond

Melatonin, often called the sleep hormone, is pivotal in regulating our sleep-wake cycle. Its production in the pineal gland is influenced by the light-dark cycle of our natural environment, with levels rising in the evening to promote sleepiness and decreasing in the morning to help wake us up. For some, especially those who struggle with sleep onset due to irregular schedules or certain disorders, supplementing with melatonin can be beneficial. It is beneficial for individuals dealing with delayed sleep phase syndrome, where the internal clock is skewed much later than the conventional sleep time, or for those experiencing jet lag due to rapid cross-time-zone travel. Melatonin supplements can help realign the body's internal clock with the external environment, facilitating easier and more restful sleep.

Beyond melatonin, there are other supplements recognized for their sleep-promoting properties. Valerian root, for example, is a herb that has been used for centuries to reduce anxiety, promote calmness, and improve sleep quality. Its effectiveness is due to its interaction with gamma-aminobutyric acid (GABA), a neurotransmitter that helps regulate nerve cells and calms anxiety. Clinical studies suggest valerian root may help people fall asleep faster and improve sleep quality.

Magnesium is another supplement with significant benefits for sleep. It plays a crucial role in supporting deep, restorative sleep by maintaining healthy levels of GABA. Magnesium can also help quiet the nervous system and prepare the body for sleep, making it an excellent supplement for those who experience restless sleep or insomnia.

L-theanine, an amino acid found in green tea, is noteworthy for its ability to promote relaxation without sedation. It works by increasing serotonin, dopamine, and GABA levels in the brain, which helps regulate emotions, mood, concentration, alertness, and sleep. L-theanine also has the unique property of reducing the jitters associated with caffeine consumption, making it beneficial for those who consume caffeine but need to manage its anxiety-inducing effects.

Following specific guidelines is crucial to ensure safety and effectiveness when using any supplement. Start with the lowest possible dose to see how your body reacts before increasing to the desired level. Timing is also important; melatonin should be taken about 30 minutes before bedtime to mimic the body's natural secretion. Always read and follow the dosage recommendations provided on the supplement packaging or as a healthcare provider advises.

Consulting with a healthcare provider before starting any supplement regimen is essential, especially if you have existing health conditions or are taking other medications. Supplements can interact with medications, have side effects, or be contraindicated for specific health issues. A healthcare provider can offer guidance based on your specific health needs and help you understand each supplement's potential benefits and risks.

Incorporating supplements into your sleep routine can be a practical component of managing sleep issues, particularly when used in conjunction with other sleep-promoting practices such as maintaining a regular sleep schedule, creating a restful sleeping environment, and managing stress. By understanding and utilizing these tools, you can take a comprehensive approach to improving your sleep, enhancing both the quality and duration of your rest.

As we conclude this exploration into the impactful world of diet, exercise, and supplements on sleep, remember that the journey to better sleep is multifaceted. It encompasses the foods you eat, your activities, and the natural and supplemental aids that prepare your body and mind for rest. Each chapter of this quest brings you closer to understanding the mechanisms behind good sleep and equips you with practical tools to achieve it. As we transition from the tangible influences of diet and exercise to the cognitive realms in the next chapter, remember that improving sleep is a balance of mind, body, and lifestyle adjustments, each supporting the other in your pursuit of restful nights and energized mornings.

Chapter Five

Mindfulness and Relaxation Techniques

As the evening shadows lengthen and the bustling noise of the day begins to taper into the tranquil whispers of night, many find themselves not in the embrace of anticipated rest but wrestling with the invisible yet palpable chains of wakefulness. During these quiet hours, the mind, unfettered by the day's distractions, often displays an array of thoughts, concerns, and anxieties, turning what should be a time of rest into a time of restlessness. What if you could turn the key to unlock a serene passage to sleep, guided not by a pharmacological solution but by the innate power of your mind? This chapter introduces mindfulness meditation, a powerful tool that can transform your pre-sleep ritual, fostering a sanctuary of calm in both mind and body and escorting you gently into the realm of sleep.

Basics of Mindfulness Meditation for Sleep

Define Mindfulness Meditation

Mindfulness meditation is an ancient practice, yet it fits seamlessly into modern life, offering a respite from the chaos often found both without and within. At its core, mindfulness is about being fully present in the moment, engaging with the here and now without judgment. This might seem simple, but it is anything but that; our minds are often tangled in past regrets or future anxieties. When applied to sleep, mindfulness becomes a tool to anchor you in the present, which is particularly useful when the mind wants to wander down the winding paths of 'what-ifs' and 'if-onlys' at night.

Guide Through Basic Meditation Techniques

To begin integrating mindfulness into your bedtime routine, start with basic techniques that encourage a focus on the breath—your natural anchor to the present moment. **Breath-focused meditation** involves observing the breath as it enters and exits the body, noting the rise and fall of your chest or the sensation of air passing through your nostrils. This practice can be done while lying in bed, helping to shift your focus away from intrusive thoughts and toward a physical sensation that embodies the present moment.

Another effective technique is the **body scan**, which can be particularly soothing as you prepare for sleep. Start at your toes, bringing your attention to any sensations you feel in that part of your body. Gradually move your focus up through each part of your body, from your feet to the crown of your head. This not only helps in grounding your thoughts in the present but also aids in relaxing each part of the body, thereby enhancing physical relaxation, which is conducive to sleep.

Discuss the Benefits for Insomnia

Research has shown that mindfulness meditation can be a potent ally against insomnia. A study published in the *Journal of the American Medical Association* found that mindfulness meditation helped reduce sleep disturbances in older adults, significantly improving sleep quality (source: JAMA). By reducing the racing thoughts and bedtime anxiety that often accompany insomnia, mindfulness can decrease sleep latency—the time it takes to fall asleep—and increase overall sleep duration. Furthermore, regular mindfulness practice can help alter sleep patterns in a lasting way, promoting more profound and more restorative sleep.

Offer Tips for Creating a Consistent Practice

Consistency is key in any mindfulness practice, especially when used to improve sleep. To make mindfulness meditation a reliable part of your evening routine, consider setting aside a specific time each night for this activity. Even just five to ten minutes can be beneficial. Create a conducive environment for meditation by ensuring your bedroom is a calm, comforting space, free from distractions like loud noises or harsh lights. You should include a brief session of gentle stretching before your meditation to prepare your body for sleep physically.

Incorporating mindfulness meditation into your nightly routine opens the door to a more serene bedtime experience. This practice prepares your mind and body for sleep and enriches your overall well-being by providing a space for daily relaxation and reflection. As you continue to explore the techniques and benefits outlined in this chapter, remember that the journey to better sleep is not just about closing your eyes to the world but about opening your mind to the present moment, finding peace within it, and letting that peace lull you into a restful slumber.

Progressive Muscle Relaxation and Deep Breathing Exercises

Progressive Muscle Relaxation (PMR) is a technique that has gained considerable attention for its ability to alleviate stress and prepare the body for a restful night's sleep. It involves a two-step process where you systematically tense and then relax different muscle groups throughout the body. This method is based on the principle that physical relaxation can promote mental calmness – crucial for those nights when sleep seems just out of reach. By deliberately tensing each muscle group and then releasing that tension, you signal to your body that it's time to relax, helping to quiet the mind and ease into sleep.

To engage in PMR, start by finding a quiet, comfortable place where you won't be disturbed. This could be your bed or a soft mat on the floor. Begin with your feet and work your way up to your face and head. For each muscle group, follow this routine: first, focus on specific muscles, such as your toes. Tense these muscles as tightly as possible, but without straining, holding this tension for about five seconds. Then, suddenly release the tension, allowing the muscles to become loose and relaxed. Take a moment to enjoy the sensation of relaxation and then move on to the next muscle group — the feet, calves, thighs, and so forth until you reach the top of your head. The key here is to isolate each muscle group as much as possible, focusing on the sensation of tension and then the contrasting sensation of relaxation. This practice helps reduce physical tension and directs your focus away from stressful thoughts that interfere with sleep.

In conjunction with PMR, deep breathing exercises are an effective tool to enhance relaxation further. One particularly useful technique is the 4-7-8 breathing method, which involves breathing in deeply for 4 seconds, holding the breath for 7 seconds, and exhaling slowly for 8 seconds. This method works by increasing the amount of oxygen in your bloodstream, slowing your heart rate, and releasing more carbon dioxide from the lungs. Start by sitting or lying in a comfortable position, ideally in the same place where you performed PMR. Close your eyes to help focus on the breathing. Place one hand on your belly and the other on your chest. As you breathe in deeply through your nose, let your belly push your hand out, keeping your chest still. Hold this breath, then exhale completely through your mouth, making a whoosh sound and letting your belly fall inward. This technique can be repeated several times, each cycle helping to calm the nervous system and reduce stress levels, making it easier to transition into sleep.

The physiological effects of PMR and deep breathing exercises on sleep are profound. Both practices activate the parasympathetic nervous system, the part of the autonomic nervous system responsible for the body's 'rest and digest' functions, instead of the 'fight or flight' responses induced by stress. Activation of the parasympathetic nervous system leads to a decrease in heart rate and blood pressure, conditions that are conducive to sleep. By lowering these physical symptoms of stress, your body can shift more smoothly into sleep mode, allowing for a night of deeper, more restful sleep.

Integrating PMR and deep breathing into your evening routine doesn't require excessive time or special equipment, making them accessible methods for anyone to improve their sleep quality. Whether you struggle to switch off after a hectic day or wake up in the middle of the night, anxious thoughts whirling through your mind, these techniques offer a practical approach to ease both body and mind into the peaceful embrace of sleep. As you continue to practice these techniques, they improve your sleep and enhance your overall relaxation and well-being during waking hours.

Visualization and Guided Imagery for Sleep

In the quiet moments before sleep, the mind often wanders through the stresses and strains of the day, replaying events or anticipating future challenges. This mental activity can be a significant barrier to falling asleep, keeping the brain engaged when it should be winding down. Visualization, or guided imagery, offers a powerful tool to redirect your mind toward a calm state, facilitating a smoother transition into sleep. This technique involves forming mental images that evoke a sense of peace and relaxation, effectively diverting your thoughts from stressors that inhibit sleep.

Visualization works by engaging the mind with positive, soothing images, thereby reducing the mental chatter that can keep you awake. For instance, imagine walking along a serene beach. Visualize the warm sand under your feet, the rhythmic sound of waves crashing gently on the shore, the soft hues of the sunset stretching across the horizon, and the gentle breeze caressing your skin. This detailed mental imagery distracts from anxiety-inducing thoughts and promotes relaxation by stimulating areas of the brain involved in emotion regulation and relaxation responses. Similarly, envisioning yourself floating on a cloud, feeling weightless and carefree, can instill a profound sense of calm that prepares your mind and body for sleep.

For those new to this practice, here's a simple guided imagery script you can try tonight: "Close your eyes and take a deep breath. Imagine yourself at the edge of a quiet forest just before sunset. As you step into the forest, you notice the path beneath your feet, covered in soft, fallen leaves. With each step, you hear the gentle rustling of the leaves, soothing like a whispered lullaby. The trees around you are tall and majestic, their leaves whispering in the gentle evening breeze. You feel the air, cooler and fresher with each breath you take. As you walk further, you come across a small clearing with a soft blanket of grass under a canopy of stars. Lie down on the grass, feeling the earth supporting you, grounding you. Look up at the sky, observing the stars twinkling like diamonds scattered across a velvet cloth. Each breath brings you deeper into a state of relaxation, and with each star you count, you feel more and more at ease, ready to drift into a peaceful sleep."

Creating your own imagery can be particularly effective, as it allows you to tailor the scenario to your personal preferences and what you find most soothing. Start by identifying environments or scenarios that evoke feelings of happiness and relaxation. It could be a place you've visited, a scene from a favorite movie, or an entirely imaginary setting. Build this scene in your mind, incorporating as many senses as possible. What do you see, hear, feel, or even smell? The more detailed the imagery, the more engaging it will be, effectively diverting your mind from stress and easing you into sleep.

Research supports the benefits of visualization, indicating that the technique can significantly reduce the time it takes to fall asleep. By creating a mental narrative that promotes relaxation, visualization decreases cognitive arousal—the state of being mentally active—which is often a barrier to sleep. Studies have shown that individuals who practice visualization regularly fall asleep faster and experience better quality sleep, waking up feeling refreshed and alert.

Incorporating visualization into your bedtime routine can transform those minutes or even hours of tossing and turning into a quick, smooth transition into sleep. This practice does not require any special equipment or conditions, making it an accessible option for anyone looking to improve their sleep quality. Whether you're struggling with occasional sleeplessness or more chronic sleep difficulties, visualization offers a gentle yet effective way to calm the mind, soothe the body, and invite the restful sleep you need to rejuvenate and restore.

Yoga and Tai Chi: Gentle Movements for Better Sleep

In the quiet hours, as dusk fades to night, your body and mind seek a peaceful transition into sleep—a transition that the ancient yoga and Tai Chi practices can beautifully support. Both forms of exercise are renowned for their physical benefits and profound ability to calm the mind and prepare the body for restful sleep. Rooted in centuries of tradition, yoga, and Tai Chi embody principles of gentle movement, breath control, and mental focus, all of which are conducive to relaxing the body and easing into a state of deep rest.

With its various styles and poses, yoga offers a flexible approach to winding down after a day. For sleep preparation, certain gentle yoga poses can be particularly effective. Poses like Balasana (Child's Pose) allow you to surrender the day's burdens as you fold forward, easing tension in the back and shoulders. Similarly, Viparita Karani (Legs Up the Wall Pose) is excellent for soothing swollen or tired legs after long hours of standing or sitting; this pose also facilitates venous drainage and increases circulation, helping to calm the body. Supta Baddha Konasana (Reclining Bound Angle Pose) is another recommended pose that opens up the chest and helps alleviate breathing difficulties, promoting better oxygen intake and, thus, better sleep.

Tai Chi, often described as meditation in motion, combines flowing movements with deep breathing and mental concentration. The gentle, rhythmic movements of Tai Chi can help reduce stress and anxiety, making it easier to achieve the mental quietude necessary for sleep. One simple Tai Chi exercise that can be performed before bed involves the practice known as 'wave hands like clouds,' where you mimic the slow, smooth movements of clouds drifting across the sky. This movement promotes a focus on fluid motion and breath, diverting your mind from daily stressors and anchoring you in the present moment.

The best time to practice these activities as part of your bedtime routine is typically in the evening, about an hour before you plan to go to bed. This timing allows you to unwind from the day's activities and signals to your body that it is time to start winding down. Creating a conducive environment for these practices is also key. Ensure your practice space is quiet, dimly lit, and free from distractions. You might play soft, ambient music or light a candle to enhance the calming atmosphere. The goal is to create a peaceful setting that facilitates relaxation and introspection.

Exploring the science behind the benefits of yoga and Tai Chi reveals their significant impact on reducing stress hormones and increasing melatonin production. The physical postures and controlled breathing in yoga stimulate the parasympathetic nervous system—the part of the autonomic nervous system responsible for the body's rest and digest functions. This stimulation helps lower cortisol levels, the body's stress hormone, and enhances melatonin production, the hormone that regulates sleep. Tai Chi, with its meditative movements, has a similar effect. It reduces the production of stress hormones and increases endorphin release, creating a sense of calm and well-being conducive to good sleep.

By incorporating these gentle, restorative practices into your evening routine, you not only enhance your physical flexibility and balance but also foster a deeper connection between mind and body. This connection is essential for managing stress and achieving a state of relaxation that is ideal for a restful night's sleep. As you continue to practice and integrate these movements into your nightly routine, you may notice an improvement in your sleep quality and overall nighttime tranquility, proving that sometimes, the best way to sleep better is not just about doing less but about moving mindfully.

The Role of Aromatherapy in Promoting Sleep

Aromatherapy, an ancient practice that harnesses the essence of plants through their oils, offers a natural pathway to enhancing physical and emotional health. These essential oils, extracted from flowers, herbs, and trees, are the backbone of aromatherapy and can be particularly effective in promoting relaxation and sleep. This form of therapy taps into the olfactory system, the body's sense of smell, which is directly connected to the limbic system, the part of the brain that regulates emotions and memory. When inhaled, the molecules of essential oils interact with this system, influencing mood and physical state, and can be particularly beneficial in the preparation for sleep.

Among the myriad of essential oils, certain ones are renowned for their sedative properties, making them ideal for inclusion in a bedtime routine. Lavender, for instance, is widely appreciated for its soothing scent and ability to decrease heart rate and blood pressure, thus setting the stage for a peaceful night's sleep. Chamomile, another popular choice, is celebrated for its calming effects on the mind and body, often used to reduce anxiety and facilitate relaxation. Bergamot, though a citrus scent, is surprisingly beneficial for sleep as it can help alleviate stress and tension. When used thoughtfully, these oils can transform your pre-sleep ritual, enveloping you in a cocoon of calm that nurtures sleep.

Incorporating these essential oils into your nighttime routine can be done in several practical ways. Using a diffuser is the most direct method, as it disperses the oil into the air, allowing for easy inhalation and continuous benefit throughout the night. Simply add a few drops of your chosen essential oil to the diffuser filled with water and let it run as you prepare for bed. Alternatively, topically applying essential oils can provide more localized benefits. Mixing a few drops of essential oil with a carrier oil, such as jojoba or sweet almond oil, and massaging it into the skin, particularly on pressure points like the wrists or temples, can be a soothing pre-sleep ritual. However, it's crucial to always dilute essential oils with a carrier oil before skin application to avoid irritation. Another method is using pillow sprays, which involve a light misting of a diluted essential oil solution onto your pillow. This method allows you to inhale the relaxing scent of the oil as you drift off to sleep.

The efficacy of aromatherapy in promoting sleep is not just anecdotal; scientific research backs its benefits. Studies have shown that inhaling lavender oil before bed helps people fall asleep more quickly and enhances sleep quality. One study published in the *Journal of Alternative and Complementary Medicine* found that participants who used lavender aromatherapy at bedtime reported higher vigor the following morning, suggesting a deeper, more restorative sleep. These findings highlight how inhaling certain scents can engage the body's natural relaxation responses, preparing it for a deep, rejuvenating sleep.

By integrating the art of aromatherapy into your bedtime routine, you create an environment that supports mind and body in unwinding and disconnecting from the day's stresses. This chapter has explored how essential oils can be a key component of this process, offering a simple yet profound method to enhance sleep quality naturally. As you continue to explore these aromatic tools, remember that the goal is to find what works best for you, creating a personalized bedtime ritual that fosters relaxation and invites sleep.

In summary, this chapter's journey through mindfulness and relaxation techniques offers a comprehensive toolkit to combat insomnia. From mindfulness meditation to the soothing scents of aromatherapy, each method uniquely enhances your nighttime routine and improves your sleep. As we transition into the next chapter, we'll explore further practical measures and lifestyle adjustments to support your quest for better sleep, ensuring that each night leads to rest, rejuvenation, and a revitalized morning.

Chapter Six

Cognitive Behavioral Therapy for Insomnia (CBT-I)

As dusk falls and the world quiets, many find themselves at the mercy of a relentless mind that refuses to settle into the night's embrace. The quest for sleep becomes a nightly ordeal, filled with frustration and anxiety about the sleep that should come but often doesn't. What if a structured, scientifically-backed approach could transform these restless nights into periods of peaceful slumber? This is where Cognitive Behavioral Therapy for Insomnia (CBT-I) comes into play, offering a proven strategy for those seeking liberation from the clutches of insomnia.

Understanding CBT-I: The Evidence-Based Approach

Cognitive Behavioral Therapy for Insomnia, commonly referred to as CBT-I, is a structured program that addresses the thoughts and behaviors that prevent you from sleeping well. It involves regular sessions with a trained therapist tailored to your specific sleep problems. Unlike sleeping pills, CBT-I helps you overcome the underlying causes of your sleep problems. The therapy is highly endorsed by leading sleep experts and health organizations worldwide, recognized for its effectiveness in treating chronic sleeplessness without the dependency risks associated with medication.

The efficacy of CBT-I is well-documented in numerous scientific studies. Research consistently shows that CBT-I significantly improves sleep in people with insomnia, often outperforming sleep medications. Most participants in these studies experience quicker times falling asleep and fewer awakenings during the night and report improved daytime functioning. For example, a landmark study published in the journal "Sleep" demonstrated that CBT-I considerably improved sleep in over 70% of participants, with benefits lasting well beyond the end of treatment.

CBT-I's holistic approach is what sets it apart from other treatments. It doesn't just focus on alleviating symptoms; it aims to modify the cognitive processes and habits at the root of insomnia. The therapy involves several components, each targeting different aspects of the sleep problem. These include sleep hygiene education, which teaches about the lifestyle and environmental factors that affect sleep, and sleep restriction therapy, which reduces the time spent in bed to match the actual sleep time, thereby consolidating sleep and increasing sleep efficiency.

A typical CBT-I program lasts about 6 to 8 weeks, with one weekly session lasting approximately 60 to 90 minutes. The first part of the therapy involves gathering detailed information about your sleep patterns and identifying the factors contributing to your insomnia. This phase sets the stage for subsequent sessions focusing on specific techniques to improve sleep. These techniques are practiced and refined throughout the therapy, with adjustments made based on your progress and feedback.

Interactive Element: Reflection Section

Take a moment to reflect on your current beliefs about sleep. Do you find yourself thinking that you won't function the next day if you don't get enough sleep tonight? Are you worried that you're losing control over your ability to sleep? Writing down these thoughts can help you identify patterns that may be addressed in CBT-I.

CBT-I offers hope for those who have long struggled with sleep, providing tools and techniques that empower you to reclaim the night and transform it from a time of stress to a time of rest. By addressing both the psychological and behavioral components of insomnia, CBT-I not only improves sleep in the short term but also equips you with the skills to maintain good sleep habits on your own. As we delve deeper into the components and benefits of CBT-I, consider how this evidence-based approach could be the key to unlocking the restful sleep that has eluded you.

Keeping a Sleep Diary: The First Step in CBT-I

Embarking on the path to better sleep through Cognitive Behavioral Therapy for Insomnia often begins with a simple yet powerful tool: the sleep diary. This essential component is not just a sleep record; it's a reflective mirror providing insights into the habits and patterns that shape your nightly rest. A sleep diary helps both you and your therapist pinpoint the specific behaviors and circumstances that contribute to your insomnia, making it a foundational element of CBT-I.

Maintaining a sleep diary involves logging daily aspects of your sleep and waking life. Critical entries include the time you go to bed, the time it takes you to fall asleep (sleep latency), the number of times you wake up during the night, the duration of these awakenings, the total sleep time, and the time you finally get up. Besides these timings, it's important to note the quality of your sleep and how you feel upon waking—refreshed or fatigued—as well as details about your daytime naps, exercise routines, and consumption of caffeine or alcohol. Each of these factors can significantly influence sleep patterns and are valuable data points for developing your treatment plan.

Let's walk through a sample sleep diary entry to understand how this data is used:

- **Bedtime:** 11:00 PM

- **Sleep Latency:** 45 minutes

- **Number of Awakenings:** 3

- **Awake Time During the Night:** 30 minutes total

- **Wake Time:** 6:30 AM

- **Total Sleep Time:** 6 hours 15 minutes

- **Perceived Sleep Quality:** Poor

- **Daytime Functioning:** Felt drowsy and had trouble concentrating

- **Other Notes:** Drank coffee at 4 PM; felt stressed about work

Analyzing this sample, several patterns might be affecting sleep quality. The late afternoon coffee could be delaying sleep onset, while stress could be contributing to awakenings during the night. This straightforward but detailed recording offers tangible targets for intervention, such as adjusting caffeine habits and incorporating stress-reduction techniques.

Understanding how the diary informs treatment is crucial. In CBT-I, this ongoing record helps both you and your therapist identify which interventions are working and which aspects of your sleep hygiene need more attention. For instance, if initial changes to your bedtime routine don't affect your sleep latency, further adjustments can be made, such as more stringent limits on screen time before bed or relaxation exercises to perform right before turning off the lights. This dynamic tool not only guides the course of your therapy but also empowers you to see the direct impact of changes to your behavior on your sleep patterns, enhancing your motivation and adherence to the therapeutic plan.

Maintaining a sleep diary might initially feel cumbersome, but its benefits are profound. This simple practice cultivates an awareness of your sleep habits and their consequences, providing you and your therapist with the information needed to tailor your treatment effectively. As you continue to record and review your sleep with your therapist, you'll likely discover insights and solutions that had previously eluded you, illuminating the path to a night of more peaceful and restorative sleep.

Restricting Sleep: A Counterintuitive Approach

At first glance, the idea of restricting sleep to combat insomnia might seem paradoxical. However, sleep restriction is a core component of

Cognitive Behavioral Therapy for Insomnia (CBT-I) and is based on a principle that may initially challenge conventional wisdom. The concept revolves around limiting the amount of time spent in bed to the actual amount of sleep obtained rather than the time spent trying to sleep. This method is designed to increase sleep efficiency—the percentage of time spent asleep while in bed. By reducing the mismatch between the time spent in bed and the actual sleep time, sleep restriction can help consolidate sleep, enhance sleep quality, and reduce the anxiety and frustration often associated with prolonged periods of wakefulness in bed.

Implementing sleep restriction typically begins with keeping a detailed sleep diary to assess your average sleep duration accurately. Let's say you generally spend 8 hours in bed but only sleep for 5. The approach would then involve limiting your bedtime to these 5 hours. While this might sound daunting, the method is not about depriving you of sleep but rather about building a stronger drive for sleep that leads to quicker sleep onset and fewer awakenings during the night. Gradually, as sleep efficiency improves, the time in bed is incrementally increased. This careful calibration helps maintain the pressure to sleep and gradually extends sleep duration.

To start, you would establish a fixed wake-up time, which is crucial for setting your biological clock. From this wake-up time, you would count backward to determine your bedtime based on the prescribed sleep window. For instance, if your wake-up time is 6:00 AM and your initial sleep window is 5 hours, your bedtime would be 1:00 AM. It is essential during this period to avoid napping, as it can decrease sleep drive and counteract the benefits of the therapy.

The adjustment period can be challenging. Common difficulties include increased sleepiness during the day and the temptation to extend sleep in the morning. However, consistency is key to success.

To manage increased sleepiness, it's advisable to engage in light, stimulating activities during the day. Strategic exposure to natural light can also help reinforce your body's circadian rhythm, enhancing wakefulness during daylight hours. If the sleepiness becomes overwhelming, a short nap in the early afternoon—no longer than 20 minutes—can be incorporated temporarily.

Case Studies: Real-Life Success Stories

Consider the experience of Jenna, a freelance graphic designer who found herself caught in a cycle of sleepless nights due to erratic work hours and chronic anxiety about sleep. After starting a sleep restriction program, Jenna initially struggled with the reduced sleep window, particularly feeling irritable and tired during the first week. However, she noticed a significant improvement as she adhered to the strict bedtime and wake-up schedule. By the second week, Jenna was falling asleep within minutes of going to bed and experiencing fewer night awakenings. Over several weeks, her sleep window gradually increased, and her sleep quality improved noticeably. Jenna's case highlights the effectiveness of sleep restriction and the importance of patience and consistency in seeing the process through.

Another example is Mark, a retired bank manager who had insomnia for several years. Mark's therapy included a sleep restriction protocol that initially limited his time in bed to 5.5 hours. Despite initial skepticism and difficulty adjusting to the shorter sleep window, Mark committed to the process. Over time, he found that not only was he sleeping more solidly during the allotted time, but he also felt more alert during the day. Mark's therapist gradually extended his sleep window, allowing more time in bed as his sleep efficiency improved. After several months, Mark regularly achieved 6.5 to 7 hours of sleep per night, a significant improvement that profoundly impacted his overall quality of life.

These testimonials underscore the potential of sleep restriction as part of CBT-I to transform sleep patterns and improve life quality. While the initial adjustment period can be challenging, the long-term benefits of increased sleep efficiency and quality can be life-changing. As you consider this approach, remember that success lies in adherence to the method and a willingness to adjust habits fundamentally. With commitment and guidance, sleep restriction can be a powerful tool in overcoming insomnia and reclaiming the restorative sleep essential for health and well-being.

Controlling Stimuli: The Association Between Bed and Sleep

Creating an environment that fosters sleep is essential, especially when struggling with insomnia. The environment where you sleep can play a critical role in how easily you fall asleep and how well you stay asleep. Various environmental factors and pre-sleep activities, known as stimulus control, can significantly influence the association between your bed and sleep. This principle lies at the heart of Cognitive Behavioral Therapy for Insomnia (CBT-I) and is centered around strengthening the connection between being in bed and sleeping.

Stimulus control is based on the idea that your bed should be a cue for sleep rather than wakefulness. This means using your bed only for sleep and intimate activities, thus avoiding activities that keep your mind alert, such as watching TV, eating, or working on a laptop. If you cannot sleep after about 20 minutes of getting into bed, it's advised to leave the bed and engage in a relaxing activity in another room. Only return to your bed when you feel sleepy. This technique helps reinforce the association between your bed and sleep, making it easier to fall asleep quickly upon going to bed.

Creating an optimal sleep environment involves more than just the right mattress or pillow—it encompasses everything from lighting to room arrangement. To enhance your sleep setting, start with lighting. Exposure to low, warm lights before bedtime can help increase your levels of melatonin, the sleep hormone, preparing your body for sleep. Consider installing dimmer switches or using lamps with warm-toned bulbs in your bedroom. On the other hand, ensure that your room can be sufficiently darkened when it's time to sleep. Blackout curtains or heavy drapes can block out street lights and early morning sunlight, which might otherwise disrupt your sleep.

Noise control is another crucial element. If you live in a noisy neighborhood or if your home has thin walls, consider using a white noise machine or earplugs to block out disruptive sounds. These devices can provide a consistent auditory backdrop that can mask interruptive noises. On the organization front, keep your bedroom tidy and clutter-free. A disorganized space can subconsciously elevate stress and distract from the calm needed for sleep. Ensure your bedroom is used primarily for rest and relaxation, not as a multipurpose room where work and leisure activities blend.

Success Stories: Transformative Changes in Sleep Environments

Take the story of Clara, a teacher who found herself regularly tossing and turning at night, her mind reeling from the day's challenges. Her bedroom was also her workspace, filled with student papers and teaching materials. Clara made significant changes after learning about stimulus control in a CBT-I session. She moved her work materials to another room, kept only a bedside lamp for soft lighting, and started using lavender-scented candles to create a calming aroma before bed. These changes transformed her sleep experience, helping her to associate her bedroom with relaxation rather than work and stress.

Similarly, consider the case of Tom, whose insomnia was exacerbated by the sounds of city traffic. Investing in soundproof windows and a high-quality white noise machine allowed him to reduce the auditory disruptions significantly. Additionally, Tom adopted a strict routine of reading a book in dim light before bedtime, avoiding screens and bright lights. These adjustments helped reinforce his bed as a place for sleep, markedly improving the speed at which he fell asleep and his overall sleep quality.

These anecdotes underscore the profound impact of modifying your sleep environment and behaviors on overcoming insomnia. By controlling the stimuli around your bedtime and sleep space, you can create a strong, positive connection between being in bed and falling asleep. This approach addresses the symptoms of insomnia and works towards a long-term solution by realigning your sleep habits and environments to support restful, uninterrupted sleep. As you consider these strategies, remember that small, consistent adjustments can lead to significant improvements, helping you transition more smoothly into restful nights.

Cognitive Restructuring: Changing Thoughts for Better Sleep

In the quiet hours of the night, as you toss and turn, the mind often plays host to a myriad of thoughts. Among these, negative thoughts about sleep can be particularly insidious, not merely disrupting a single night's rest but potentially developing into chronic insomnia. Cognitive restructuring, a core technique in Cognitive Behavioral Therapy for Insomnia (CBT-I), targets these disruptive thoughts. The technique is designed to identify, challenge, and replace negative thoughts with more balanced and realistic ones, thereby reducing anxiety and improving sleep.

Cognitive distortions about sleep are surprisingly common. You might catch yourself thinking, "If I don't get eight hours of sleep tonight, I'll ruin my presentation tomorrow," or "I'm going to have another terrible sleep tonight, just like always." Such thoughts are examples of catastrophizing and overgeneralizing, respectively—patterns of thinking that not only heighten sleep-related anxiety but also reinforce poor sleep habits. These distorted thoughts create a feedback loop where anxiety about sleep leads to increased wakefulness at night, which in turn feeds back into the anxiety, perpetuating the cycle of insomnia.

Cognitive restructuring involves several steps, beginning with identifying the negative thoughts. This might occur through discussions during therapy sessions or self-monitoring thoughts during bedtime. Once these thoughts are identified, the next step is to challenge their accuracy. This involves questioning the evidence for these thoughts, considering alternative explanations, and assessing the likelihood of worst-case scenarios. For instance, questioning how often a lack of sleep has genuinely 'ruined' a presentation could help you realize that while you might feel tired, you still perform adequately.

Replacing these negative thoughts involves formulating more balanced and rational responses. Instead of thinking, "I'll ruin the presentation," a more balanced thought could be, "I might be tired, but I'm well-prepared for the presentation." This reframing helps reduce anxiety by adjusting the emotional response to the thought, making it less likely to impact your ability to fall asleep.

Hypothetical Scenario: Cognitive Restructuring in Action

Imagine Sarah, a software developer who struggles with recurring thoughts of, "I must get perfect sleep, or I can't function." During a CBT-I session, her therapist helps her break down this thought. They explore the evidence, revealing that Sarah feels sluggish after poor nights but has never failed to meet her work deadlines. They then work on a replacement thought: "It's ideal to have good sleep, but I can manage even when I'm less rested." Over time, Sarah learns to integrate this new perspective, noticing a decrease in her bedtime anxiety and improved sleep quality.

Cognitive restructuring is not about denying insomnia's difficulties but viewing sleep in a more balanced light. This can significantly reduce the pressure and anxiety surrounding sleeping. By transforming the way you think about sleep, you enhance your ability to fall asleep and improve your overall approach to challenges, making you more resilient.

As this chapter closes, we reflect on the powerful tools CBT-I offers. By understanding and adjusting our thoughts, maintaining a sleep diary, strategically managing our sleep times, and controlling our sleep environment, we equip ourselves with robust strategies against insomnia. These tools do more than just promise a good night's rest—they empower us to transform our nights from a time of struggle to a time of peace.

The next chapter will explore additional behavioral techniques that complement the cognitive strategies discussed here, offering further means to enhance your sleep and overall well-being.

Chapter Seven

Special Considerations in Insomnia Management

As the evening sky darkens and a hush falls over the world, many find themselves not gently drifting into sleep but wrestling with the sheets, victims of insomnia's stubborn grip. While this challenge cuts across the entire spectrum of age and gender, women often face unique hurdles in their quest for restful sleep, mainly due to the ebb and flow of hormonal changes throughout their lives. This part of the book delves into how these hormonal fluctuations during the menstrual cycle and menopause can shape sleep patterns and explores tailored strategies to navigate these challenges, ensuring that sleep, an essential pillar of health, is not beyond reach.

Insomnia in Women: Menstrual Cycle and Menopause Considerations

Examining Hormonal Fluctuations and Their Impact on Sleep

For many women, the journey through the phases of the menstrual cycle and into menopause is often accompanied by varying sleep challenges. Hormones such as estrogen and progesterone, which see-saw throughout these stages, play significant roles in reproductive health and sleep regulation. During the menstrual cycle, progesterone, known for its sleep-promoting qualities, rises in the post-ovulation phase, often bringing about better sleep in the days leading up to menstruation. Conversely, the drop in progesterone along with estrogen just before menstruation can disrupt sleep, leading to difficulty in falling and staying asleep.

Menopause brings its own set of challenges as estrogen and progesterone levels decline. Estrogen is linked with regulating the sleep cycle and helps maintain REM sleep. Its reduction during menopause can lead to shorter sleep times, increased awakenings at night, and less restful sleep. Additionally, the decrease in estrogen can exacerbate sleep-disordered breathing, a condition more commonly known during menopause as obstructive sleep apnea, which disrupts the sleep cycle and diminishes sleep quality.

Discussing Common Sleep Disturbances During Menstruation and Menopause

The days preceding menstruation can often be marked by a phenomenon known as premenstrual insomnia, characterized by difficulty falling asleep and staying asleep. This type of insomnia is largely due to the sharp decline in progesterone and estrogen. Similarly, hot flashes, a hallmark symptom of menopause, can cause significant sleep disturbances. These sudden feelings of heat can lead to sweating and discomfort, abruptly waking women from sleep and making it difficult to return to slumber.

Offering Targeted Lifestyle and Dietary Adjustments

Specific lifestyle and dietary adjustments can be particularly beneficial to combat these hormonal challenges and promote better sleep. Incorporating magnesium-rich foods like leafy greens, nuts, and seeds into the diet can help enhance sleep quality. Magnesium supports deep sleep by maintaining healthy levels of GABA, a neurotransmitter that promotes relaxation and good sleep. Vitamin E, found in foods like almonds, spinach, and sweet potatoes, may also help reduce the severity of hot flashes, minimizing their impact on sleep.

Stress-reduction techniques such as yoga, meditation, and deep breathing exercises are especially useful during these times. They help manage stress that can exacerbate sleep difficulties and contribute to overall well-being, creating a more conducive state for restful sleep.

Suggesting Medical Interventions When Necessary

While lifestyle and dietary changes are crucial, they may need to be increased sometimes. In such cases, it is advisable to consult healthcare professionals who can provide guidance on hormone replacement therapy (HRT) or other medical treatments. HRT can help stabilize hormone levels, alleviating many of the menopausal symptoms that interfere with sleep. However, it's important to carefully consider this option, discussing potential benefits and risks with a qualified healthcare provider.

Understanding and addressing the unique challenges faced during the menstrual cycle and menopause is crucial to navigating the intricate relationship between hormonal changes and sleep. By tailoring strategies to these specific needs, it is possible to mitigate the impact of hormonal fluctuations on sleep, paving the way for more restful nights and vibrant, energetic days.

Aging and Sleep: Adjusting to the Needs of Older Adults

As we gracefully age, our sleep architecture, or the structure of our nightly rest, undergoes significant modifications. These changes are not just a mere inconvenience; they are profound shifts that can affect our health, mood, and daily functioning. Typically, older adults experience a decrease in deep sleep, the most rejuvenating stage. There's an increase in the lighter stages of sleep, which are far less restorative. This shift can often lead to waking up and not feeling refreshed, even after adequate sleep hours. Additionally, the circadian rhythms that regulate our sleep-wake cycles adjust as we age, often leading to earlier bedtimes and wake times. This shift, known as advanced sleep phase syndrome, can disrupt an individual's social life and lead to frustration and isolation.

In the realm of sleep disorders, certain conditions become notably more prevalent as we grow older. Sleep apnea, a disorder characterized by pauses in breathing or shallow breaths during sleep, tends to increase in frequency and severity with age. This condition not only disrupts sleep but also poses serious risks to cardiovascular health. Another common issue is restless legs syndrome (RLS), a neurological disorder that causes uncomfortable sensations in the legs and an irresistible urge to move them. These sensations typically occur in the evening or during periods of inactivity, such as when lying in bed. RLS can severely disrupt sleep and, by extension, impair quality of life.

Adjustments to the sleep environment and bedtime routines are often necessary to address these age-related changes and disorders. For instance, adapting the bedroom to enhance comfort and safety can make a significant difference. Installing night lights can prevent falls during nocturnal bathroom trips, a common issue for many older adults. Similarly, choosing a supportive mattress and pillows can help alleviate discomfort from conditions like arthritis, which worsens at night and disrupts sleep. Tailoring the bedtime routine to align with the body's adjusted circadian rhythm is also beneficial. Engaging in relaxing activities such as reading or listening to soft music can ease the transition to sleep, accommodating the body's tendency to sleep and wake earlier.

Regular medical check-ups become increasingly important as we age, not only for general health but also for maintaining good sleep. Conditions like arthritis, prostate or bladder issues, and cardiovascular diseases can significantly impact sleep quality. For example, the frequent need to urinate at night, known as nocturia, is common in older men with prostate issues and in women who have experienced menopause. This condition can severely disrupt sleep architecture, leading to fragmented sleep patterns that prevent deep, restorative sleep. Sleep quality can be markedly improved by managing these underlying health issues through regular medical consultations and treatments.

In addressing the sleep needs of older adults, it becomes clear that a proactive approach, one that adapts to the body's changing requirements, is essential. This approach enhances the quality of nightly rest and supports overall health and well-being, allowing for a more vibrant and fulfilling lifestyle even as we age. Adjusting sleep environment routines and addressing medical issues are all steps toward respecting and aligning with the natural aging process, ensuring that sleep, a critical component of life, is not left by the wayside as we age.

Insomnia and Coexisting Health Conditions

When night falls and the world quiets, the quest for sleep begins—a quest that, for many, is complicated by health conditions that intertwine intricately with insomnia. Understanding these relationships is crucial, not just for managing sleep but for overseeing overall health. Conditions such as chronic pain, diabetes, and cardiovascular diseases frequently coexist with insomnia, each capable of disrupting the delicate balance of sleep and significantly impacting life quality.

Chronic pain, for instance, is a pervasive ailment that affects a substantial portion of the population, with profound implications for sleep. Pain can make finding a comfortable position challenging, leading to prolonged sleep onset times and frequent awakenings at night. This disruption in the sleep cycle can prevent the deep, restorative sleep needed to manage pain effectively, creating a cycle where pain leads to sleep loss, leading to increased pain sensitivity. Similarly, diabetes influences sleep through various pathways. Fluctuations in blood sugar levels can lead to changes in sleep patterns, with high blood sugar causing frequent urination that disrupts sleep. Low blood sugar can potentially lead to night sweats or even nighttime awakenings. Moreover, the stress and anxiety associated with managing diabetes can further complicate sleep, making it harder to fall and stay asleep.

Cardiovascular diseases also share a bidirectional relationship with sleep. Conditions like hypertension and heart disease can be worsened by sleep deprivation, which in turn may exacerbate these conditions. Poor sleep can lead to higher blood pressure, increased heart rate, and inflammation, all risk factors for cardiovascular disease. Sleep apnea, a disorder characterized by repeated breathing interruptions during sleep, is commonly associated with cardiovascular problems and can lead to a fragmented sleep pattern that diminishes sleep quality and increases nighttime blood pressure.

Addressing these co-morbid conditions requires a holistic approach considering each condition's direct and indirect effects on sleep. Managing chronic pain, for instance, may involve a combination of medication, physical therapy, and cognitive-behavioral strategies to reduce pain intensity and improve sleep. Techniques such as guided imagery, mindfulness meditation, or gentle nighttime yoga can help ease the mind and body, making it easier to fall asleep despite pain. For managing diabetes, stabilizing blood sugar levels is paramount. This might involve dietary adjustments, medication, and perhaps most crucially, regular monitoring of blood sugar levels to prevent the peaks and troughs that disrupt sleep. Establishing a bedtime routine that includes checking blood sugar levels can help prevent nighttime disturbances and provide peace of mind, promoting better sleep.

Lifestyle modifications that also improve sleep can enhance cardiovascular health. Regular physical activity, a balanced diet, and weight management are crucial, as are stress-reduction techniques and adequate sleep hygiene practices. For those with sleep apnea, continuous positive airway pressure (CPAP) therapy can significantly improve sleep quality and cardiovascular health by stabilizing breathing during sleep.

The role of interdisciplinary care in managing these complex interactions cannot be overstated. Collaborating with various healthcare providers—from physicians and dietitians to physical therapists and sleep specialists—is essential for developing a comprehensive treatment plan that addresses the symptoms and the underlying causes of sleep disturbances. This collaborative approach ensures that all aspects of a person's health are considered, providing a unified strategy to improve sleep and overall well-being.

For anyone navigating the complexities of insomnia alongside other health conditions, understanding these interconnections and adopting an integrated approach to treatment can make a significant difference. By addressing the health conditions that influence sleep while simultaneously implementing strategies to improve sleep directly, it's possible to enhance both nighttime rest and daytime vitality, breaking the cycle of sleeplessness and its associated health challenges. This holistic view improves sleep and empowers individuals to manage their health proactively, embracing a healthier, more rested life.

Shift Work and Irregular Schedules: Strategies for Adaptation

In the stillness of night, while much of the world lies sleeping, a significant portion of the workforce is clocking in. For those engaged in shift work, the unconventional hours are more than a mere inconvenience; they represent a fundamental challenge to the body's internal clock or circadian rhythm. This rhythm, an internal mechanism synced mainly with the natural light-dark cycle of our environment, dictates not just sleep but also various physiological functions.

Working non-traditional hours, such as overnight shifts or rotating schedules, disrupts this natural rhythm, often leading to shift work sleep disorder (SWSD). This disorder is characterized by insomnia when sleep is desired, wanted, or needed and excessive sleepiness while awake. The symptoms not only degrade sleep quality but also impact overall health and quality of life, manifesting in both physical tiredness and cognitive declines, such as reduced alertness and impaired decision-making.

One of the most effective strategies to combat the effects of SWSD involves managing light exposure to realign the circadian rhythm with work demands. Light is the most powerful cue for shifting the phase of the circadian clock, signaling when to wake up and when to sleep. Exposure to bright light during the shift can help promote alertness for night shift workers. Devices like light boxes or special glasses that emit bright, blue light can simulate daylight, tricking the body into a wakeful state. Conversely, minimizing exposure to light when it's time to sleep is crucial. This can be achieved by using blackout curtains or eye masks to create a dark sleeping environment and avoiding blue light from screens at least an hour before bedtime.

Supplemental use of melatonin can also be beneficial for shift workers. Melatonin supplements can help induce sleep when taken at the right time, aiding in quickly adjusting the body's internal clock to align with a new sleep schedule. However, timing is critical—the supplement should be taken about 30 minutes before the desired sleep time, after a night shift, to cue the body that it's time to wind down. It's important to note that melatonin should be discussed with a healthcare provider to ensure it's appropriate based on individual health needs and other medications.

Adjusting sleep habits is equally crucial for mitigating the effects of irregular schedules. Strategic napping can be a significant asset; a nap before starting a night shift can reduce sleepiness during work, while a short nap during breaks can help maintain alertness. However, the length of naps is vital—long naps can lead to sleep inertia, a state of grogginess and disorientation that can occur upon waking from deep sleep. Ideally, naps should be kept between 20 to 30 minutes. Maintaining a consistent sleep schedule, even on days off, is another critical strategy. While it's tempting to revert to a more conventional sleep schedule during off days, this can further disrupt the circadian rhythm. Sticking as closely as possible to the same sleep schedule helps maintain the body's internal clock, reducing the degree of circadian misalignment.

The workplace's role in supporting shift workers' health and sleep cannot be overstated. Employers have a crucial role in scheduling practices that minimize circadian disruption. Implementing forward-rotating shifts, where the worker moves from a morning to an afternoon to a night shift, can be less disruptive than backward rotation. Providing well-timed breaks during shifts can also help manage fatigue, allowing workers the opportunity to rest and recuperate. Workplaces that prioritize their employees' sleep health enhance their workforce's well-being and benefit from higher productivity and reduced errors, underscoring the mutual benefits of well-considered scheduling practices.

Shift work, with its inherent challenges to sleep and health, requires a proactive approach to manage effectively. Shift workers can mitigate the impact of their irregular hours by strategically using light exposure, melatonin supplementation, napping, consistent sleep schedules, and supportive workplace policies. These adaptations improve sleep quality and enhance overall health and job performance, providing the tools needed to thrive despite the challenges of non-traditional work hours.

Travel and Jet Lag: Managing Sleep Across Time Zones

When you cross multiple time zones, your body's internal clock, or circadian rhythm, which dictates sleep-wake cycles along with other physiological functions, struggles to align with the local time. This misalignment results in jet lag, a temporary sleep disorder marked by insomnia, general fatigue, and even digestive problems. The severity of jet lag directly correlates with the number of time zones crossed; the more significant the change, the more pronounced the symptoms. This disruption occurs because the cues that usually reset our circadian rhythms, primarily light exposure, suddenly don't match the internal time our body is programmed to follow.

Adjusting your sleep schedule before you travel can be incredibly beneficial in easing the transition across time zones and mitigating the effects of jet lag. Start by gradually shifting your bedtime and wake-up time closer to the schedule of your destination. If you're traveling east, go to bed one hour earlier each night for a few nights before departure. For westward travel, do the opposite by staying up later. This gradual shift can help ease the adjustment once you arrive, making the transition less jarring.

Exposure to natural light is also a powerful tool for resetting your circadian clock. If you're heading east, seek morning light at your destination, which will help advance your body clock. Conversely, if you're traveling west, exposure to late afternoon sunlight can help delay your body clock to align better with the new time zone. These adjustments in light exposure can significantly help in reducing the severity of jet lag symptoms and speed up the adjustment process.

When traveling, managing sleep on the go is crucial. Selecting flights that align with your natural sleep schedule can help; for example, choosing a night flight if you sleep well on planes or a day flight if you don't, allowing you to stay awake and adjust more quickly to the new time zone upon arrival. If sleep aids are necessary, use them sparingly and preferably under the guidance of a healthcare provider. Over-the-counter options like melatonin, taken in small doses, can aid sleep at the right time according to the new time zone, helping to reset your internal clock more swiftly.

Creating a conducive sleep environment in hotels or guest accommodations is also key. Portable sleep aids such as eye masks, earplugs, and travel pillows can help recreate the comfort of your home sleep environment, making it easier to fall and stay asleep. Additionally, maintaining a bedtime routine similar to the one at home can provide a sense of familiarity and prompt your body to prepare for sleep, even in a new environment.

Recovering from jet lag doesn't end with the right preparation and on-the-go strategies; it also involves specific practices once you reach your destination or return home. To realign your circadian rhythm, manage light exposure by spending plenty of time outdoors during daylight hours. Keep a consistent sleep schedule, go to bed and wake up at the same time every day, and avoid naps outside of these times, especially long ones, as they can make adjusting to the new time zone harder.

This approach to managing sleep while traveling across time zones minimizes the discomfort of jet lag and enhances your overall travel experience, allowing you to be more alert and enjoy your new surroundings. Whether it's a business trip that demands peak performance or a vacation for some much-needed relaxation, understanding, and managing jet lag is key to making the most of your time away from home.

As we close this discussion on navigating sleep while traveling, it's clear that with the right strategies, the challenges of jet lag can be effectively managed, ensuring that your adventures across time zones leave you enriched rather than exhausted. Moving forward, the focus will shift from addressing specific sleep challenges to exploring the future of sleep technology and innovations that continue transforming how we understand and manage sleep in our fast-paced, globally connected world. By staying informed and proactive, you can harness these advancements to enhance your sleep quality and overall well-being wherever you are in the world.

Chapter Eight

Advanced Techniques and Therapies

As the curtain of night falls, countless individuals find themselves caught in a silent battle against restlessness, their minds and bodies unwilling to succumb to sleep. If you've ever felt held hostage by your alertness, longing for the escape of slumber, you understand the profound desire for new solutions. This chapter invites you to explore the innovative realm of biofeedback—a technique that stands on the cutting edge of sleep therapy, offering a bridge between the conscious and unconscious workings of your body.

Biofeedback and Sleep: Listening to Your Body's Signals

Biofeedback is about gaining insight into your physiological processes and learning to modulate them through conscious control. This technique utilizes sensors attached to your body to measure functions like heart rate, brain waves, and muscle tension, which are typically automatic and not under voluntary control. These measurements are fed back to you in real-time via signals on a monitor, allowing you to observe and learn how to influence these functions. The ultimate goal is to harness this awareness to induce relaxation and improve health conditions, including those that affect sleep.

Biofeedback can be particularly transformative for individuals battling insomnia, especially when stress and anxiety are the culprits. Two specific types of biofeedback have shown promise in this area: EEG biofeedback, commonly known as neurofeedback, and heart rate variability (HRV) biofeedback. Neurofeedback focuses on the brain's electrical activity. By monitoring brain wave patterns, individuals can learn to promote calming and relaxation patterns that are conducive to sleep. For instance, increasing theta wave activity through neurofeedback has been linked to improved sleep quality, as these waves are prevalent during light stages of sleep and are thought to contribute to the relaxation necessary for deeper sleep stages.

HRV biofeedback, on the other hand, measures the time interval between heartbeats, which varies as you breathe in and out. Lower variability indicates stress and sympathetic nervous system activation, while higher variability is associated with relaxation and parasympathetic response. By using HRV biofeedback, you can learn to control your breathing and enhance heart rate variability, which promotes a state of calmness and facilitates the onset of sleep.

Numerous studies support the efficacy of biofeedback in improving sleep. Research has demonstrated that both forms of biofeedback can significantly reduce the time it takes to fall asleep and increase total sleep time, particularly in individuals whose insomnia is linked to anxiety or stress. For example, a study published in the journal

'Applied Psychophysiology and Biofeedback' found that individuals who underwent HRV biofeedback sessions showed marked improvements in sleep quality and a reduction in anxiety, suggesting that this technique not only helps in managing insomnia but also addresses some underlying causes of sleep disturbances.

If you're considering biofeedback as a solution for your sleep issues, the first step is to find a qualified practitioner. Biofeedback therapy should be conducted by a certified professional who can ensure the correct use of the equipment and guide you through the process effectively. Typically, biofeedback therapy sessions last about 30 to 60 minutes, with the total number of sessions required varying based on individual needs. Most people see benefits after eight to ten sessions, though some may notice improvements earlier.

Getting Started with Biofeedback

To embark on biofeedback therapy, consult your healthcare provider for referrals or search for certified practitioners through reputable sources like the Biofeedback Certification International Alliance (BCIA). During your first session, the therapist will explain the process, place sensors on specific areas of your body, and start recording the physiological activities that will guide your training. The key to success with biofeedback is consistency and practice; the more you engage with the process, the better you will become at controlling your physiological responses and, consequently, improving your sleep.

As you explore biofeedback, remember that this technique is part of a broader approach to managing insomnia. It can be incredibly effective when combined with other treatments and lifestyle changes, such as cognitive behavioral therapy for insomnia (CBT-I), proper sleep hygiene, and relaxation techniques. Integrating biofeedback into your sleep improvement plan opens up a new dimension of possibilities for achieving the restful nights that have seemed just out of reach.

Hypnosis for Sleep: An Underutilized Resource

In the quiet hours of the night, when sleep should be most welcoming, you might find yourself caught in the frustrating grip of insomnia. Amid the various therapies and treatments available, hypnosis stands out as a profound yet often overlooked tool that can significantly enhance your sleep quality. Hypnosis, by definition, is a state of heightened focus and concentration, usually accompanied by deep relaxation. This state is achieved with the help of a trained therapist who uses verbal repetition and mental images to lead you into this trance-like state. Despite common misconceptions, hypnosis is not about being put into a deep sleep or losing control over your actions; instead, it's a therapeutic tool that facilitates powerful mental relaxation and focus, which can be directed toward improving sleep patterns.

The mechanisms by which hypnosis aids sleep are deeply rooted in its ability to alter states of consciousness. When you're hypnotized, the therapist can implant suggestions that help in reducing thoughts that commonly lead to anxiety or stress, both of which are significant barriers to sleep. For instance, through hypnosis, you can learn to redirect your focus from stress-inducing thoughts to more calming imagery or sensations, effectively lowering mental agitation and preparing your mind for sleep. This mental shift is crucial because it decreases sleep onset latency—the time it takes to fall asleep—and reduces nocturnal awakenings, thus enhancing the continuity and quality of sleep.

Clinical studies have consistently underscored the effectiveness of hypnosis in managing sleep disorders. Research published in the

'Journal of Clinical Sleep Medicine' found that participants who underwent hypnosis reported quicker sleep onset and longer duration of deep sleep compared to those who didn't use hypnosis. These benefits were particularly pronounced in individuals who were considered highly susceptible to hypnotic suggestions, highlighting the importance of a personalized approach in the use of hypnosis for sleep improvement.

Finding a qualified hypnotherapist is crucial to safely and effectively using hypnosis for sleep enhancement. It's important to look for practitioners who are certified in hypnotherapy and have specific training and experience in dealing with sleep disorders. Certified practitioners can be found through professional bodies such as the American Society of Clinical Hypnosis (ASCH), which provides a directory of licensed therapists. When you start therapy, you can expect sessions to typically last between 60 and 90 minutes, with the number of sessions needed varying based on your specific circumstances and the severity of your insomnia.

How to Begin Hypnotherapy for Sleep

To initiate hypnotherapy, first have a detailed discussion with your therapist about your sleep patterns, any underlying issues you might be facing, and what you hope to achieve through hypnosis. This initial conversation sets the foundation for tailored sessions addressing your needs. During hypnosis, the therapist will guide you into a relaxed state and then introduce positive suggestions and guided imagery that promote sleep. These suggestions are designed to take effect both during the session and after you return to your normal daily activities, gradually helping to alter your sleep habits and reduce insomnia.

Incorporating hypnotherapy into your sleep improvement plan offers a unique opportunity to tap into the power of the mind-body connection. By engaging with this technique, you open yourself up to a transformative experience that enhances sleep and contributes to overall stress reduction and well-being. As you continue to explore advanced techniques for managing insomnia, remember that treatments like hypnosis provide not just a remedy for sleep disturbances but a pathway to deeper, more restorative sleep, unlocking a night of peace that has seemed just out of reach.

The Promise of Light Therapy in Regulating Sleep Cycles

As you lie in bed, enveloped by darkness, your body's internal clock—the circadian rhythm—tells you it's time to rest. Yet, the signal doesn't seem strong enough for many, and sleep remains elusive. Light, the natural regulator of our circadian rhythms, plays a pivotal role in signaling when it's time to wake up and when to wind down. Understanding this, imagine harnessing light as a therapeutic tool to realign these rhythms and encourage better sleep. This is the essence of light therapy, a treatment that uses exposure to specific types of light to stimulate changes in the body's sleep-wake cycles.

Light therapy involves using devices such as light boxes or wearable devices emitting light, mimicking natural sunlight. These tools are not just about illumination; they are carefully designed to produce light at specific wavelengths that trigger biological processes in the body. For instance, exposure to light in the blue wavelength range has been shown to suppress melatonin production, the hormone that helps regulate sleep and wake cycles. By timing this exposure, light therapy can shift your circadian rhythms forward or backward, helping to reset your internal clock to a more desired schedule.

For those wrestling with insomnia, particularly when it involves difficulty falling asleep at a conventional bedtime, light therapy offers a beacon of hope. The key to its effectiveness lies in the timing, duration, and intensity of light exposure. To advance a delayed sleep phase, which keeps you awake late into the night, exposure to bright light in the morning can help shift your sleep pattern earlier. This morning light exposure helps reset the circadian clock, promoting earlier melatonin production in the evening, which can facilitate an earlier bedtime. Conversely, if you find yourself waking too early, exposure to light in the early evening can help delay your sleep phase, allowing you to sleep longer into the morning.

While light therapy is powerful, it's not without considerations and precautions. The intensity of the light, the duration of exposure, and the specific timing during the day are all critical factors that need to be tailored to individual needs. Typically, light therapy sessions can range from 20 to 60 minutes and may vary in duration depending on the individual's response to the treatment and the specific condition being addressed. It's also important to consider the potential side effects. For some, exposure to bright light, especially later in the day, can lead to difficulty falling asleep or potential mood changes. Furthermore, for individuals with certain eye conditions or those taking medications that increase light sensitivity, light therapy may not be suitable or may require close supervision by a healthcare provider.

If light therapy sounds like a suitable approach for you, starting involves a few steps. First, it's advisable to consult with a healthcare provider or a sleep specialist who can assess your specific sleep issues and recommend a light therapy regimen that fits your needs. They can guide you on using the devices properly and safely, ensuring you gain the maximum benefit without exacerbating sleep issues or negatively impacting your mood. Many modern light therapy devices are designed for ease of use and can be used at home, making them a convenient option for regular use.

By integrating light therapy into your routine, aligned with guidance from a sleep specialist, you can harness the natural power of light to realign your biological clock. This alignment can facilitate a more regular sleep schedule, ease the transition to sleep, and enhance the overall quality of your rest. Whether you're struggling with falling asleep too late, waking up too early, or dealing with jet lag fatigue, light therapy provides a method to recalibrate your internal rhythms, using the natural influence of light to foster better nights and more vibrant mornings.

Therapeutic Sound and Music Therapy for Sleep

Imagine the soft hum of a distant fan or the rhythmic cadence of rain tapping against the window—sounds often accompanying the descent into sleep's embrace. This innate connection between sound and relaxation forms the foundation of sound therapy, a therapeutic approach that leverages auditory stimuli to enhance sleep quality and alleviate disorders such as insomnia. Sound therapy encompasses a range of techniques, each designed to soothe the mind, reduce stress, and foster a deep, restorative sleep.

At the heart of sound therapy is the principle that certain sounds can significantly influence our mental state and physiological responses, particularly those related to relaxation and stress reduction. White noise machines are among the most popular and effective forms of sound therapy, which produce a consistent, ambient sound that masks disruptive background noises that might prevent or disrupt sleep.

These devices are particularly beneficial in noisy environments, where street sounds or household noises can intrude upon the silence that sleep demands. The consistent hum of white noise provides a kind of sonic blanket, enveloping you in a sound that calms the mind and reduces the likelihood of sleep disturbances.

Another innovative form of sound therapy involves binaural beats, which play two slightly different frequencies in each ear. The brain perceives these as a single tone that fluctuates at the difference of the frequencies, which is believed to encourage brainwave frequencies associated with relaxation. For example, suppose a frequency of 300 Hz is played in one ear and 310 Hz in the other. In that case, the brain will process a 10 Hz binaural beat, promoting relaxation and potentially enhancing the depth and quality of sleep.

Therapeutic music playlists designed specifically for sleep are another tool in the sound therapy arsenal. These playlists often feature slow, rhythmic melodies and are structured to gradually slow your heart rate and breathing, guiding you naturally toward sleep. The tempo and rhythm of the music are typically aligned with the relaxed state of the heart rate, which can help facilitate the onset of sleep and improve the duration of deep sleep.

A variety of studies supports the effectiveness of sound therapy. Research indicates that sounds like white noise or binaural beats can significantly reduce the time it takes to fall asleep. Moreover, these sound therapies have decreased the frequency of nocturnal awakenings, thereby improving the continuity and quality of sleep. For instance, a study published in the Journal of Sleep Medicine & Disorders found that participants who listened to white noise showed improved sleep continuity and decreased sleep onset latency, highlighting the potential of sound therapy as a powerful tool for those struggling with sleep disturbances.

Incorporating sound therapy into your sleep routine can be a simple yet effective way to enhance your sleep environment and quality. When choosing sound therapy tools, consider the specific issues you face with sleep. For instance, a white noise machine might be particularly beneficial if household noises easily awaken you. If anxiety or a racing mind is keeping you awake, then binaural beats or a therapeutic music playlist might be more effective. Setting up an effective auditory environment for sleep involves more than just playing sounds; it requires creating a space where these sounds can be calming. Ensure your sleeping area is comfortable and free from distractions, and set the volume to an audible level but not overpowering.

By integrating sound therapy into your nightly routine, you create an atmosphere conducive to sleep that not only quiets the external environment but also soothes the internal chaos of stress or anxiety. As you explore the nuances of this therapy, remember that the goal is to find the sounds that resonate best with your personal sleep needs, using them as tools to unlock the restorative power of sleep each night.

Acupuncture and Acupressure for Insomnia Relief

In the stillness of the night, when the world slows, and the mind should follow, many find themselves grappling with the elusive pursuit of sleep. If you are among those who twist and turn, watching the shadows change, you might find ancient solutions like acupuncture and acupressure particularly intriguing. Rooted in Traditional Chinese Medicine (TCM), these practices are built on the principles of energy flowing through pathways in the body known as meridians. These meridians are thought to be conduits for the life force or Qi. According to TCM, the proper flow of Qi is essential for health, and disruptions in this flow can lead to issues like insomnia.

Acupuncture involves the insertion of thin needles into specific points along these meridians, which is believed to restore the balance and flow of Qi. Acupressure, conversely, does not involve needles but uses gentle to firm finger pressure on the same points. Both techniques aim to release tension, promote relaxation, and stimulate the body's healing processes. For those battling insomnia, these treatments offer a pathway to calm the nervous system and encourage the body to prepare for sleep more naturally and effectively.

The effectiveness of acupuncture and acupressure in treating insomnia is not just anecdotal; several scientific studies lend credence to these practices. Research has shown that acupuncture can increase the secretion of nocturnal melatonin, a hormone that regulates sleep patterns, and significantly improve total sleep duration. Moreover, it's been found to reduce anxiety, which is often a significant component of insomnia. Acupressure, too, is effective in improving sleep quality, especially in individuals who prefer a non-invasive approach to their sleep troubles. One study published in the Journal of Sleep Medicine demonstrated that participants who received acupressure treatments over weeks reported faster sleep onset and decreased wakefulness during the night.

If this approach to managing insomnia appeals to you, finding a qualified practitioner is essential. Acupuncturists and acupressure therapists should be certified and have specific training in handling sleep-related issues. It's advisable to consult with a practitioner who has credentials and a good understanding of sleep dynamics. During your initial visit, expect a detailed discussion about your sleep patterns, lifestyle, and overall health. This holistic view allows the practitioner to tailor the treatment to your specific needs.

Treatments typically last from 20 to 60 minutes, and the number of sessions needed can vary based on the individual's response to the treatment. Many find relief after just a few sessions, while others may need ongoing sessions to maintain the benefits. Acupuncture and acupressure are often part of a broader approach that may include herbal medicine, dietary changes, and exercise recommendations, all aimed at optimizing your body's energy flow and enhancing your ability to sleep well.

As you consider this ancient yet dynamic approach to overcoming insomnia, remember that the goal is to rebalance your body's energies and enable a natural transition to sleep. While the night may stretch long, the relief found in the precise touch of acupuncture or the steady pressure of acupressure is the key to reclaiming your night's rest. As you explore these options, you engage not just with a treatment but with a tradition that views sleep not as a mere physical necessity but as a critical element of your body's harmony and balance.

Technology to Help with Sleep

In your quest for a deeper, more restorative sleep, technology offers innovative solutions catering to various aspects of sleep enhancement. From the soothing hum of white noise machines to the insightful data provided by smart sleep trackers, these tools harness the power of modern technology to create optimal environments and habits for better sleep.

White Noise Machines

Imagine a device that effortlessly masks the jarring sounds of urban life or the irregular disturbances in your home, enveloping your bedroom in a cocoon of soothing sound. White noise machines do just that, utilizing a consistent sound frequency to create a calming atmosphere that promotes easier onset and maintenance of sleep. These devices are not limited to mere 'white noise'—they often include a variety of soundscapes, such as rain, ocean waves, or forest sounds, which you can choose based on your personal preference. The key benefit lies in their ability to drown out distracting noises that disrupt your sleep cycle, making them especially valuable in noisy environments. By maintaining a steady, calming background noise, these machines can help reduce the time it takes to fall asleep and help you stay asleep by minimizing the disruptive impact of sudden sound disturbances.

Smart Sleep Trackers

Transitioning to a more analytical approach, smart sleep trackers represent a significant advancement in sleep technology. Wearable devices like smartwatches and fitness bands go beyond tracking physical activity and have evolved to provide detailed insights into your sleep patterns. These devices comprehensively analyze your sleep stages and cycles by monitoring movements, heart rate, and even respiratory rates throughout the night. This data is invaluable as it allows you to understand how long and how well you sleep, highlighting periods of restlessness or waking that you might not be aware of. Many sleep trackers also offer gentle wake-up alarms, which rouse you during your lightest sleep phase, making waking up less jarring. Some devices include guided breathing exercises that help you relax and wind down before bed, further enhancing your ability to fall asleep naturally and peacefully.

Blue Light Blocking Glasses

In the age of screens, our exposure to blue light has dramatically increased, and its effects on sleep are notably disruptive. The blue light emitted by smartphones, tablets, and computers can interfere with the production of melatonin, the hormone that signals to our bodies that it's time to sleep. Here's where blue light-blocking glasses come into play. By filtering out blue light in the hours leading up to bedtime, these glasses help maintain your natural circadian rhythm, making it easier to wind down and prepare for sleep. For those who use electronic devices in the evening, whether for winding down with a movie or catching up on emails, wearing blue light-blocking glasses can be a simple yet effective way to mitigate the sleep-disrupting effects of screen time.

Smart Lighting Systems

Expanding the role of light in sleep enhancement, smart lighting systems like Philips Hue offer a dynamic solution. These systems can be programmed to mimic the natural progression of sunlight throughout the day, gradually dimming and changing hues to encourage relaxation as nighttime approaches. By providing a visual cue to your body's internal clock, or circadian rhythm, these lights help prepare your physiological state for sleep. As the lights dim, they signal to your body that it's time to produce melatonin, thus promoting a natural onset of sleepiness. This can be particularly beneficial for establishing a consistent sleep schedule, reinforcing the natural cues that trigger sleepiness at the right time.

Sleep Meditation Apps

Lastly, the digital realm offers sleep meditation apps, which have become popular for many seeking a non-pharmacological solution to sleep difficulties. Apps like Calm and Headspace provide a variety of guided meditations, bedtime stories, and soothing soundscapes designed to help you relax and drift off to sleep. These apps are particularly useful for those whose insomnia is driven by stress or anxiety, as the guided meditations focus on relaxation techniques that can ease the mind and prepare the body for sleep. With user-friendly interfaces and customizable features, these apps make it easy to incorporate meditation into your nightly routine, offering a practical way to enhance your sleep quality through relaxation and stress reduction.

As we conclude this exploration of technological advancements in sleep assistance, it's clear that these tools offer a range of solutions tailored to different needs and preferences. From soundscapes that shield you from disruptive noises to devices that analyze and improve your sleep patterns, technology has harnessed a variety of ways to enhance our sleep experience. Integrating these tools into your sleep routine can address specific sleep challenges and enhance your overall sleep quality, making restful nights more attainable and mornings more refreshing. The next chapter will delve into the psychological dimensions of sleep as we move forward, exploring how our mental states interact with our sleep patterns and how we can manage these influences to enjoy better sleep.

Chapter Nine

Building Resilience and Maintaining Sleep Health

As dusk falls and the world quiets, the quest for peaceful slumber begins. Yet, for many, this quest is often fraught with difficulty. The delicate dance of drifting into sleep is not just about closing one's eyes and hoping for the best—it's about crafting the right environment both internally and externally. In this chapter, we focus on nurturing resilience and fostering a sustainable environment that encourages restorative sleep. Here, we explore the foundational aspect of recognizing healthy sleep, understanding its characteristics, and appreciating its profound impact on your daily life.

Recognizing Healthy Sleep

Healthy sleep is the cornerstone of physical well-being and emotional and psychological health. It is more than the absence of insomnia—it is the presence of rest that rejuvenates, refreshes, and restores. Recognizing healthy sleep involves understanding its structure, quality, and effects on day-to-day functioning.

The Structure of Sleep

Sleep architecture refers to the cycle of sleep phases that occur at night, from light to deep sleep and REM (Rapid Eye Movement) sleep. Each stage plays a crucial role in health and recovery. For instance, deep sleep aids in physical recovery and immune function, while REM sleep, often associated with dreaming, supports memory consolidation, emotional regulation, and problem-solving skills. A healthy sleep pattern, without frequent awakenings, includes smooth transitions between these stages and aligns with the body's natural circadian rhythms, promoting optimal hormonal balance and bodily functions.

Quality Over Quantity

While the duration of sleep is important, quality often trumps quantity. Quality sleep means falling asleep within a reasonable time after getting into bed (typically within 20 minutes), not waking up frequently during the night, and feeling rested upon waking in the morning. It's possible to spend 8 hours in bed but only achieve a few hours of quality sleep, which can be just as detrimental as outright sleep deprivation. The depth and restfulness of your sleep are crucial indicators of its quality.

Impact on Daily Life

The effects of healthy sleep extend far beyond the hours spent in bed. Good sleep enhances cognitive functions such as concentration, memory, and decision-making. It also improves emotional resilience, helping you manage stress and react more calmly in challenging situations. Physically, quality sleep is linked to lower risks of chronic conditions like hypertension, diabetes, and obesity. It bolsters the immune system, making you less susceptible to infections and quicker to recover when ill.

Recognizing Sleep Issues

It is vital to recognize the signs that indicate your sleep lacks quality. Symptoms such as daytime drowsiness, difficulty concentrating, mood swings, or a reliance on caffeine to get through the day can all suggest inadequate sleep. By paying attention to these signs, you can take proactive steps to assess and improve your sleep habits.

Interactive Element: Sleep Quality Assessment Checklist

To help you evaluate your sleep quality, consider the following questions:

- Do you often take more than 30 minutes to fall asleep?
- Do you frequently wake up during the night?
- Do you feel groggy or fatigued during the day?
- Do you rely on sleep aids or alcohol to fall asleep?
- Do you feel irritable or anxious due to poor sleep?

If you answer "yes" to any of these questions, it may be time to examine your sleep habits more closely and consider strategies for improvement. These could include adjusting your sleep environment, revisiting your pre-bedtime routine, or consulting a sleep specialist.

Understanding and recognizing healthy sleep is just the first step in building a resilient approach to sleep health. By appreciating the nuances of what makes sleep restorative and recognizing the early signs of sleep disturbances, you can make informed decisions that enhance your sleep quality and, by extension, your overall health and well-being. As we continue to explore the elements of building resilience in sleep health, remember that each small step you take can significantly improve how you sleep and live.

Developing a Proactive Sleep Mindset

Adopting a proactive sleep mindset is fundamental to achieving and maintaining healthy sleep, especially for those who frequently find themselves awake when they desperately wish to be asleep. This proactive approach involves anticipating sleep challenges and implementing strategies to mitigate them before they escalate into more severe issues. It's about shifting from a reactive stance—where actions are taken only after problems arise—to one of prevention and regular maintenance. By cultivating this mindset, you prepare yourself to improve the quantity and quality of your sleep and enhance your overall health and well-being.

A proactive sleep mindset starts with cultivating sleep positivity. For many, especially those battling insomnia, sleep can become a source of anxiety and frustration. Negative feelings and dread about going to bed can exacerbate sleep difficulties, creating a self-fulfilling prophecy where worry about sleep leads to increased sleeplessness. To counter this, it's important to foster positive attitudes towards sleep. This can be achieved by focusing on the benefits of good sleep rather than the consequences of poor sleep. Remind yourself of how refreshing and invigorating a good night's sleep feels and its positive impact on your energy levels, mood, and productivity. Consider keeping a sleep gratitude journal where you note down positive sleep experiences or how you felt after a good night's sleep, reinforcing the benefits and creating a positive association with going to bed.

Encouraging active participation in sleep hygiene is another cornerstone of a proactive sleep mindset. Sleep hygiene encompasses various practices that are conducive to better sleep. This includes establishing a regular sleep schedule where you go to bed and wake up at the same time every day, which helps regulate your body's internal clock. Creating a pre-sleep routine that promotes relaxation is equally important. This might involve activities such as reading, taking a warm bath, or practicing relaxation exercises like progressive muscle relaxation or deep breathing techniques. It's also crucial to optimize your sleep environment—ensure your bedroom is dark, quiet, and cool and that your mattress and pillows are comfortable and supportive. By consistently engaging in these practices, you actively contribute to the likelihood of a good night's sleep.

Integrating mindfulness throughout the day also plays a pivotal role in cultivating a mindset conducive to sleep. Mindfulness involves maintaining a moment-by-moment awareness of our thoughts, feelings, bodily sensations, and the surrounding environment. It's particularly effective in reducing stress and anxiety, which are common culprits behind sleep disturbances. Practicing mindfulness can help you manage the stressors of daily life more effectively, preventing them from overwhelming you at night. Techniques such as mindful breathing or taking short mindful breaks during the day can help lower stress levels and lead to a calmer state of mind by bedtime. Furthermore, mindfulness can enhance your ability to disconnect from the incessant flow of thoughts that may impede sleep, allowing for a smoother transition to sleep.

By nurturing a proactive sleep mindset, you take control of your sleep health, using preventive measures and regular maintenance to foster a restful night. Remember, each small, positive decision you make regarding your sleep hygiene and daily stress management adds up, paving the way toward more peaceful nights and energized days. As you continue to apply these principles, you'll find that your sleep and overall quality of life improve.

Regular Check-Ins: Monitoring Your Sleep Health

Understanding your nightly patterns plays a pivotal role in improving sleep. It's not merely about achieving a certain number of hours of sleep but about grasping the quality and rhythm of those sleeping hours. To this end, various tools and technologies have been developed to assist you in tracking your sleep, providing insightful data that can help you make informed adjustments to your sleep habits. From traditional sleep diaries to modern wearable devices and mobile apps, these tools offer a window into your nocturnal life, shedding light on what happens when you close your eyes each night.

A sleep diary is a simple yet effective tool for tracking sleep. It involves recording details about your sleep habits, such as the time you go to bed, how long it takes you to fall asleep, the number of times you wake up during the night, your wake-up times, and how rested you feel in the morning. Over time, this record can reveal patterns and triggers that affect your sleep quality, such as the impact of caffeine or alcohol consumption, stress, and even exercise habits. For example, consuming coffee late in the afternoon correlates with difficulty falling asleep or that exercising in the evening leads to a more restful night.

In the age of technology, wearable devices like fitness trackers and smartwatches have added a layer of convenience and precision to sleep tracking. These devices use sensors to monitor your movements and heart rate throughout the night, distinguishing between different sleep stages, such as light, deep, and REM sleep. Many also measure other physiological markers like respiratory rate and body temperature, which can provide clues about your sleep health. Mobile apps linked to these devices can offer a user-friendly interface where you can view trends over time, receive personalized insights, and even get suggestions for improving your sleep.

When interpreting sleep data, it's important to focus on trends rather than isolated incidents. Look for changes in sleep duration, quality, and disturbances over extended periods. This can help you identify if a particular intervention—like a change in your bedtime routine or a new mattress—has a positive effect. It's also beneficial to pay attention to how changes in your daytime activities, such as increased stress or changes in diet, may impact your sleep. This holistic view can help you understand how interconnected your daily life and sleep patterns are.

Textual Element: Tips for Adjusting Sleep Plans Based on Data

Once you have gathered and reviewed your sleep data, consider the following guidelines to adjust your sleep environment and routines:

- **Consistency is Key**: To regulate your body's internal clock, try going to bed and waking up at the same time every day.

- **Optimize Your Sleep Environment**: Ensure your bedroom is conducive to sleep—consider temperature, noise, and light factors. Experiment with adjustments and note any improvements in your sleep data.

- **Mind Your Diet and Exercise**: Look for patterns linking your eating and exercise habits to your sleep quality. Adjust timing and types of meals and workouts based on your findings.

- **Manage Stress**: If data shows you sleep poorly on more stressful days, incorporate stress-reduction techniques like meditation or deep breathing into your routine.

Maintaining a regular schedule for monitoring your sleep can provide many benefits. It allows you to see the effects of lifestyle changes, understand the factors contributing to good or poor sleep, and make ongoing adjustments to enhance your sleep quality. Over time, this proactive approach can significantly improve your sleep and, by extension, your overall health and well-being. Remember, the goal of regular sleep monitoring is not just to gather data but to use this data to create a healthier, more balanced lifestyle that supports restful nights and energetic days. By staying informed and responsive to your body's needs, you empower yourself to take control of your sleep health, leading to a more vibrant and productive life.

When to Seek Professional Help: Signs and Guidance

Navigating the complexities of sleep disturbances can sometimes feel like a solitary journey, but it's important to recognize when to seek the guidance of a professional. While self-management strategies are

THE INSOMNIA BREAKTHROUGH: 113

effective for many, there are instances where they need to be more. If you find yourself struggling with persistent insomnia despite your best efforts, or if your sleep issues begin to impede your daily activities significantly, it may be time to consult with a sleep specialist. This step is not about admitting defeat but taking control of your health and well-being with expert support.

Recognizing when professional intervention is needed is crucial. Key indicators include the frequency and duration of sleep issues and their impact on your daily life. If you notice that lack of sleep is affecting your ability to function—perhaps you're feeling unusually irritable, finding it difficult to concentrate at work, or more prone to accidents—it's a sign that your sleep problems may require more than lifestyle adjustments. Additionally, if your nights are frequently haunted by severe anxiety about sleep or if you find yourself waking up gasping for air or experiencing unsettling phenomena like sleep paralysis, these are strong cues to seek professional advice.

The next step is understanding the types of professionals who can help with sleep issues. Sleep disorders are complex and can be approached from different angles. Sleep physicians are medical doctors who specialize in diagnosing and treating sleep disorders through methods such as sleep studies, medical treatments, and lifestyle advice. Psychologists or psychiatrists specializing in sleep disorders can provide cognitive behavioral therapy for insomnia (CBT-I), which helps address the thoughts and behaviors affecting your sleep. They can also help manage any underlying mental health issues, such as anxiety or depression, that might be contributing to your sleep problems.

Preparing for a sleep consultation is essential to maximize your visit. Documenting your sleep patterns through a sleep diary is incredibly helpful. This should include details such as when you go to bed and wake up, how long it takes you to fall asleep, how often and why you wake up at night, and how you feel in the morning. Additionally, bringing a list of any medications you are taking and a summary of your medical history can provide valuable insights for the specialist. Be ready to discuss any previous treatments for insomnia you have tried, including over-the-counter and prescription medications, as well as any other therapies.

During the consultation, the sleep specialist might suggest various interventions based on your specific condition. Participating in a sleep study may be necessary to diagnose issues such as sleep apnea. For others, CBT-I might be recommended to address behavioral aspects of insomnia. Medication may also be considered, particularly if your insomnia is severe and other treatments have not been effective. It's important to discuss the potential benefits and side effects of any treatment thoroughly with your specialist to make an informed decision that aligns with your health goals and lifestyle.

Navigating the path to better sleep sometimes requires professional guidance, and recognizing when to seek this help is crucial in managing your sleep health effectively. By understanding the signs that indicate the need for professional intervention and preparing adequately for consultations, you can take proactive steps toward restoring restful nights and vibrant days.

Joining Support Groups and Communities

In the gentle quiet of the night, while many find solace in their dreams, others find themselves wrestling with the elusive shadow of sleep. If you are one of those who frequently count more sheep than hours of sleep, the journey towards restful nights can sometimes feel lonely and daunting. However, it's important to remember that you're far from being alone in this experience. Support groups and communities dedicated to sleep health can offer a sanctuary of shared experiences and collective wisdom. Engaging with these groups provides emotional support and practical advice that can be transformative in managing insomnia.

Support groups, whether online or in person, serve as invaluable resources for individuals grappling with insomnia. They offer a platform to share experiences, tips, and encouragement in a nonjudgmental setting. The feeling of isolation that often accompanies sleep disorders can be significantly alleviated when you realize there are others who understand precisely what you are going through. These communities foster a sense of belonging and can be a wellspring of emotional support and empathy, which is crucial when dealing with the stress and frustration that sleep deprivation brings.

Beyond emotional support, these groups can also be a great source of practical advice. Members often share what has or hasn't worked, from the latest sleep hygiene techniques to recommendations for sleep aids and adjustments to daily routines. This pooling of collective knowledge can provide you with new strategies and insights into what might best suit your situation. Moreover, many support groups are facilitated by health professionals who can offer expert guidance and debunk common myths about sleep, ensuring that the information shared is accurate and beneficial.

Finding the right support group might seem challenging, but numerous resources are available. Many hospitals and health centers host sleep disorder support groups that meet regularly. Additionally, the internet has made accessing support more accessible than ever. Online forums and social media platforms like Facebook and Reddit host myriad groups focused on sleep health. Websites dedicated to sleep education often have links to both local and virtual support groups. For instance, the American Sleep Association and similar organizations provide directories of support groups in person and online, ensuring you can find a community regardless of location.

Participation in community events and workshops focused on sleep education is another avenue through which valuable support and information can be accessed. These events provide educational resources and opportunities to connect with others facing similar challenges, broadening your support network. Health fairs, sleep health workshops, and seminars conducted by sleep specialists are common in many communities. These gatherings are beneficial for sharing information and motivating the community to engage in activities focused on improving sleep health.

Success Stories: The Impact of Community Support

To illustrate the positive impact of these support systems, consider the experience of Emma, a graphic designer who struggled with chronic insomnia for years. Feeling at her wit's end, she joined a local sleep disorder support group on the recommendation of her therapist. Through her interactions in the group, she learned about sleep restriction therapy, a method she hadn't tried before. With support from her group and guidance from her health provider, she implemented this strategy and saw a significant improvement in her sleep quality. Emma's story underscores the practical benefits of support groups and the emotional resilience from being part of a community that understands and supports her journey.

Similarly, a retired school teacher, Tom, found solace and solutions through an online forum dedicated to sleep health. Living in a rural area, there were other options than in-person groups. The online community became his go-to resource, where he could share his experiences and learn from others anytime. It was through this platform that Tom was introduced to the concept of cognitive behavioral therapy for insomnia (CBT-I), which he pursued with the help of a specialist. The improvements in his sleep profoundly affected his overall health and well-being, demonstrating the far-reaching benefits of community support in managing insomnia.

These stories highlight the transformative power of support groups and communities in sleep health. They provide a forum for sharing and learning and a collective strength that can inspire and empower individuals to take control of their sleep health. Whether through emotional support that eases the stress of sleepless nights, practical tips that pave the way for better sleep, or the camaraderie that comes from shared experiences, these communities play a crucial role in the journey towards restful nights and rejuvenated mornings.

Celebrating Sleep Successes and Setting New Goals

In the quiet victory of a night well-slept, there lies a profound sense of achievement. For those who have wrestled with the shadows of insomnia, each peaceful night is a milestone worthy of celebration. Recognizing and celebrating these victories, no matter how small, can significantly bolster your motivation and reinforce the positive momentum you've built. It's essential to take a moment to acknowledge the progress you've made on your path to better sleep. This could be as simple as noting a week where you consistently managed to go to bed at the same time or recognizing a night when you felt particularly refreshed upon waking. These moments of recognition serve as powerful affirmations of your efforts and their tangible results.

Setting realistic and achievable goals for your sleep health is crucial in maintaining this progress. Goals provide direction and purpose, turning the abstract desire for 'better sleep' into concrete targets to strive for. When setting these goals, specificity is key. Instead of vaguely aiming to 'sleep better,' set a clear, measurable objective like 'extend nightly sleep from 6 to 7 hours consistently'. Such specificity makes your goals more tangible and allows you to track your progress more effectively. Start with small, incremental changes that feel manageable. This could mean adjusting your bedtime by 15 minutes earlier each week until you reach your desired schedule. Remember, the journey to improved sleep is a marathon, not a sprint; setting too ambitious goals too quickly can lead to frustration and setbacks.

Maintaining the gains you've achieved requires a dynamic approach. As your lifestyle changes, so too might your sleep needs. Periodically revisiting and adjusting your sleep goals ensures they align with your current life circumstances and continue supporting your sleep health. For instance, if you start a new job that requires an earlier start, adjusting your bedtime routine to accommodate this change helps sustain the quality of your sleep. Additionally, continue to engage in practices that have proven effective for you, whether that's mindfulness exercises before bed, maintaining a consistent sleep schedule, or using relaxation techniques. Consistency in these practices supports ongoing sleep improvements and builds resilience against potential sleep disruptions.

Speaking of resilience, it's important to prepare for setbacks in your sleep health. Fluctuations in sleep quality are normal and can be influenced by various factors like stress, illness, or even changes in the weather. When setbacks occur, view them not as failures but as opportunities to strengthen your resilience. Evaluate what might affect your sleep and consider what adjustments could be made to mitigate these effects. Perhaps a stressful week at work has thrown your sleep schedule off balance; recognizing this link can help you focus on stress management to restore sleep quality. Keeping a positive outlook during these times is crucial; remember that progress is often non-linear, and patience with yourself is a vital part of the process.

You create a sustainable framework for long-term sleep health by celebrating each step forward, setting goals thoughtfully, and maintaining the practices that support your sleep. Each night of restful sleep builds upon the last, gradually painting a bigger picture of improved health, mood, and overall quality of life. As you continue implementing the strategies discussed in this chapter, remember that each small success is a building block to a more rested and vibrant existence.

As this chapter concludes, we've explored how recognizing achievements in sleep, setting thoughtful goals, maintaining effective practices, and building resilience can profoundly impact your journey toward sustained sleep health. This holistic approach enhances your nights and enriches your days, bringing more clarity, energy, and joy into every aspect of your life. Moving forward into the next chapter, we will delve into the exciting future of sleep health, exploring cutting-edge research, emerging technologies, and innovative practices that continue to push the boundaries of what we understand about sleep. This journey is about overcoming insomnia and embracing a lifestyle that celebrates and prioritizes restful, rejuvenating sleep.

Chapter Ten

Future Trends and Innovations in Sleep Science

As night blankets the sky and the world quiets, the silent battle for sleep begins anew for many. But what if the battleground of sheets and pillows could become a place of peace, tuned to the rhythms of your own body? This vision is fast becoming a reality with the advent of wearable sleep technology. In this chapter, we explore how these devices, once mere trackers of our daily steps, have evolved into sophisticated tools for enhancing sleep, offering personalized insights and interventions that promise to transform our nights.

The Next Frontier: Wearable Sleep Technology

Wearable technology has journeyed from simple pedometers to complex systems that monitor and analyze every heartbeat, breath, and twitch we make while we sleep. The evolution of these devices mirrors our deepening understanding of sleep's complexities and its critical role in our health. Modern wearables now offer more than just sleep duration tracking; they provide a window into the intricate dance of sleep stages, heart rate variability, and respiratory patterns. These devices, equipped with sensors and powered by advanced algorithms, paint a detailed picture of our nightly rest that was once accessible only in sleep laboratories.

The innovations in wearable sleep technology are inspiring. Imagine a device that tracks your sleep and adjusts your bedroom environment to improve it. Current developments include wearables that can control smart home systems adjusting room temperature or lighting based on real-time sleep stage data. Some devices now use artificial intelligence to learn from your sleep patterns, predicting when you might have a restless night and suggesting interventions like a guided breathing exercise or a change in your sleep schedule. These smart devices represent a leap toward a future where technology proactively supports our health, adapting to our individual needs in real time.

The role of wearables in personalized sleep analysis is pivotal. By gathering data night after night, these devices allow for a tailored approach to sleep management. They enable users to understand how various factors—such as diet, exercise, stress, and environment—affect their sleep. This data can be invaluable to the individual and healthcare providers who can use it to spot trends, diagnose disorders, and customize treatment plans. In essence, wearable technology empowers you to become an expert in your sleep, equipped with concrete data to back up the subjective experience of a good or bad night's rest.

Looking ahead, the potential future developments in wearable sleep technology are boundless. We are on the cusp of seeing devices that could directly influence sleep architecture—the fundamental structure of sleep itself. Innovations might include wearables that can emit subtle frequencies to enhance slow-wave sleep or use gentle vibrations to prevent prolonged periods of wakefulness without disturbing sleep. Integration with smart home systems could also advance further, where your wearable device communicates with your home to create the optimal environment for sleep based on your personal physiological data.

Reflective Journaling Prompt

As we contemplate these advancements, take a moment to reflect on what features would most enhance your sleep. What aspects of your sleep do you wish you had more control over? Jot these thoughts down in a sleep journal. This exercise is not just hypothetical—your current needs and desires can guide you in choosing the right technology to support your sleep now and in the future.

In this era of rapid technological advancement, the night is no longer a time to hope for rest passively but a period we can actively enhance with the right tools. Wearable sleep technology stands at the forefront of this revolution, offering new ways to reclaim the night, turning our struggles into solutions, and transforming our understanding of what a good night's sleep can look like.

Genetic Research and Personalized Sleep Medicine

As you settle into the evening, consider for a moment the profound role your genetic makeup plays in shaping your sleep patterns. The field of genetics reveals that the way we sleep, including our predisposition to disorders like insomnia, is not merely a matter of habit or environment but can also be deeply rooted in our DNA. Recent advances in genetic research have begun to uncover the links between our genes and our sleep behaviors, providing fascinating insights that could revolutionize how we approach sleep disturbances.

Genetics influence various aspects of our sleep—from the duration we need to feel rested to our susceptibility to sleep disorders and how we respond to environmental sleep disruptors. For instance, variations in genes such as DEC2 are known to affect sleep duration, with certain mutations allowing some individuals to feel fully rested after only six hours of sleep, a trait that would be desirable to many. Similarly, genes like APOE, which has several variants, have been linked to the risk of developing conditions such as sleep apnea. Understanding these genetic influences does more than satisfy academic curiosity; it opens the door to personalized sleep medicine, a field that tailors sleep interventions to an individual's genetic profile.

The advancements in genetic testing are pivotal in this respect. New technologies now allow us to identify specific genetic markers associated with sleep disorders through simple tests that can be carried out with a saliva sample. These tests can determine an individual's genetic susceptibility to insomnia, circadian rhythm disorders, and other sleep-related issues. For example, a person with a variation in the PER3 gene might be predisposed to delayed sleep phase disorder. In this condition, the individual's internal clock is shifted later than the societal norm. With this knowledge, interventions can be more accurately targeted, potentially increasing their effectiveness.

Fueled by these genetic insights, personalized sleep medicine is set to transform how we treat sleep disorders. Imagine a scenario where, based on your genetic makeup, you are prescribed a specific type of light therapy optimized for your circadian rhythm or given a customized diet plan that aligns with your metabolic needs for better sleep. This approach enhances the effectiveness of treatments and minimizes the trial-and-error process that so many endure in their quest for better sleep. It represents a shift from a one-size-fits-all approach to one finely tuned to each individual's unique genetic blueprint.

However, with these advancements come significant ethical and privacy considerations. The management of genetic data is a topic of intense debate. How do we ensure that this deeply personal information remains secure? Who has access to it, and how might it be used beyond the scope of improving sleep? The field of sleep medicine must navigate these questions carefully, establishing stringent protocols for data protection and handling. Transparency with patients about how their genetic information will be used, stored, and shared is crucial to maintaining trust and integrity in the doctor-patient relationship. Additionally, there is a broader concern about genetic discrimination, particularly regarding insurance coverage and employment. Legislations like the Genetic Information Nondiscrimination Act are steps in the right direction, but continuous vigilance is necessary to keep pace with technological advancements.

As we continue to untangle the complex web of genetics and sleep, the promise of truly personalized medicine becomes clearer. This burgeoning field can enhance our understanding of why we sleep the way we do and revolutionize the treatment of sleep disorders, making well-rested nights more accessible to all. By embracing these advancements and carefully considering their broader implications, we pave the way for a future where sleep solutions are as unique as our DNA, tailored to help each of us achieve the best possible night's rest.

Innovations in Sleep Architecture and Design

As the night deepens and you prepare to retreat into the comfort of your bedroom, consider this: the design of your sleeping environment can significantly impact the quality of your rest. Recognizing the environment's crucial role in sleep health, architects and designers

THE INSOMNIA BREAKTHROUGH:

increasingly focus on creating spaces that foster good sleep. This trend towards sleep-friendly design is reshaping private residences and the broader architectural landscape, integrating cutting-edge research into the walls surrounding us each night.

Modern sleep-centric architecture goes beyond aesthetic appeal, focusing on functional designs that enhance sleep quality. Beds and lighting systems, for example, are being reimagined with sleep in mind. Consider the evolution of the bed, traditionally a simple piece of furniture, which is now being designed with integrated technologies that adjust firmness based on body weight and sleeping position or even gently rock to enhance the deep sleep stages. Lighting systems in bedrooms are also becoming more sophisticated, equipped with technology that regulates brightness and color based on time of day, syncing with your natural circadian rhythms to promote wakefulness in the morning and relaxation in the evening.

The materials and color schemes used in bedrooms are selected based on their ability to create a calm and relaxing atmosphere. Research has shown that certain colors, such as soft blues, greens, and lavender, have a calming effect on the mind and can help lower heart rate and blood pressure, making falling asleep easier. Moreover, the bedrooms' layout is designed to minimize noise and light disruptions. Architects strategically place windows and use soundproof materials in walls to shield sleepers from the external chaos of the outside world, creating a serene oasis that encourages deep, uninterrupted rest.

These design innovations are not just for the select few; they are becoming more mainstream as awareness of sleep health grows. Furniture companies are partnering with sleep scientists to create products that are comfortable and conducive to good sleep. Retailers are beginning to feature sleep-centric design more prominently, offering products that promise to enhance sleep quality through scientifically backed design principles. This shift responds to growing consumer demand for environments that support health and wellness, reflecting a broader recognition of sleep's essential role in overall well-being.

The integration of technology and design in sleep-friendly environments is expected to increase. We can anticipate homes where sleep technology is seamlessly integrated into every element of the bedroom—from adjustable beds that track sleep health metrics to walls that change color to create the optimal environment for sleep. These advancements will likely become standard features in new housing developments, transforming our living spaces into tailored sleep sanctuaries that adjust to our individual needs.

As we embrace these changes, it's clear that the future of architectural design is not just about creating visually pleasing or functionally efficient spaces. It's about designing environments that actively contribute to health and wellness, with sleep at the forefront of this movement. The bedroom of the future will be a dynamic space, equipped not just to accommodate our sleep needs but to enhance them actively, harnessing the power of design to transform how we rest each night.

Current, Highly Regarded Sleep Health Aids

In the quest for restful sleep, technology offers innovative solutions that track sleep patterns and enhance sleep quality. Among these, the Oura Ring is a premier example of how wearable technology can seamlessly integrate into daily life to provide profound insights into your sleep health. This smart ring, designed with precision, goes beyond mere sleep tracking; it dives deep into the nuances of your sleep cycles, heart rate variability, body temperature, and overall sleep quality. By capturing a comprehensive spectrum of data through its sensors, the Oura Ring offers you a detailed analysis through its companion app. This allows you not just to understand but also to optimize your sleep patterns. The data provided can help you recognize patterns or habits disrupting your sleep, enabling you to make informed adjustments. For instance, you might discover that your deepest sleep occurs earlier at night, which could encourage you to adjust your bedtime to maximize restorative sleep. Thus, The Oura Ring serves as a monitoring tool and a personal sleep consultant, guiding you towards habits that bolster your sleep health and, by extension, your overall well-being.

Transitioning to another innovative tool, the Eight Sleep Pod, this device transforms your bed into a smart sleeping environment. Unlike traditional mattress pads, the Eight Sleep Pod is equipped with advanced technology that regulates the temperature of your bed, dynamically adjusting it through the night to sync with your sleep stages and personal comfort preferences. Temperature regulation is critical to sleep quality, as a cooler body temperature is generally conducive to better sleep. The Pod's ability to preemptively adjust the temperature based on your sleep cycle phases means you will likely experience less wakefulness and more consistent, deep sleep. Additionally, this smart mattress cover collects data on sleep metrics like heart rate variability and sleep stages, which can be accessed via an app. This feature allows you to track your sleep trends over time, providing insights into how changes in your environment or habits affect your sleep quality. The Eight Sleep Pod is crucial in promoting a deeper, more restorative sleep by ensuring you remain comfortable throughout the night and providing data-driven insights.

Another significant advancement in sleep technology is the Muse Headband, which taps into the power of meditation to enhance sleep quality. Recognizing that a calm and focused mind is essential for good sleep, the Muse Headhead uses EEG technology to monitor brain activity and provides real-time feedback during meditation. This feedback helps guide you into deep relaxation, optimal for transitioning to sleep. The headband's sensors detect your brain's activity levels and use gentle audio cues to help you refocus and deepen your meditation if your mind wanders. This real-time guidance can be particularly beneficial for those who find it difficult to settle their thoughts at night. By training your brain to reach and maintain a relaxed state more efficiently, the Muse Headband facilitates quicker sleep onset and contributes to a higher quality of sleep. It effectively bridges the gap between technology and traditional meditation practices, making it a valuable tool for anyone looking to enhance their mental relaxation and, by extension, their sleep health.

As we wrap up this exploration of current, highly regarded sleep health aids, it becomes clear that technology plays a pivotal role in tracking and actively enhancing our sleep. By embracing these innovative tools, from the Oura Ring's detailed sleep analysis and the Eight Sleep Pod's temperature regulation to the Muse Headband's meditation assistance, you are equipped to tackle the challenges of sleeplessness with advanced solutions. These technologies offer more than convenience; they provide personalized insights and interventions that make achieving restful, restorative sleep a more attainable goal.

In the next chapter, we will explore how integrating these and other technologies into everyday life continues to evolve, offering new strategies and solutions that promise to revolutionize our approach to sleep health.

Conclusion

As we draw the curtains on our comprehensive exploration of insomnia, its profound impacts, and the myriad strategies for its effective management, I would like to thank you for joining me on this enlightening journey. From the initial chapters, where we defined insomnia and delved into its various impacts on health and daily life, through the middle sections, where practical and diverse strategies were discussed, to the final chapters introducing the latest innovations in sleep science, we have traversed a landscape rich with insights and actionable knowledge.

Reflecting on our journey, it is clear that while insomnia poses a formidable challenge, it is not insurmountable. The core message of this book has been to emphasize that, with a proactive approach and the right set of strategies, you can manage insomnia effectively. Resilience, positivity, and a willingness to adapt are your greatest allies in this endeavor. Each page of this book aims to empower you with the knowledge to understand your sleep patterns and equip you with tools to enhance your nightly rest.

The key takeaways from our discussions include recognizing insomnia triggers, understanding the pivotal role of sleep hygiene, and the importance of creating a conducive sleep environment. We also touched upon the transformative potential of cognitive behavioral therapy and the promising horizon of sleep technology that personalizes your journey toward better sleep.

Now, I encourage you to take action. Take the advice and resources in this book to achieve deeper, more restorative sleep. Start with small, manageable changes to your sleep hygiene. Consider setting a regular bedtime, reducing evening screen time, and introducing relaxation techniques before bed. As you grow more comfortable, gradually incorporate more advanced strategies, tailoring them to your needs.

Please make sleep a priority and set specific, achievable goals. A practical first step could be maintaining a sleep diary, which can provide invaluable insights into your sleep patterns and highlight areas for improvement. This simple tool can be a gateway to understanding and mastering your sleep environment and routines.

Thank you for allowing me to accompany you on this journey to reclaim your nights. While each of you may face unique challenges in managing insomnia, the potential for improving your sleep and overall well-being is universal. The strategies and insights shared here will guide you to restful, rejuvenating sleep.

Here's to nights filled with peaceful sleep and days of vitality and joy.

References

National Heart, Lung, and Blood Institute. (n.d.). What is insomnia? Retrieved from https://www.nhlbi.nih.gov/health/insomnia

Stepanski, E. J., & Wyatt, J. K. (n.d.). Use of sleep hygiene in the treatment of insomnia. Retrieved from https://www.med.upenn.edu/cbti/assets/user-content/documents/Stepanski%20and%20Wyatt%20Sleep%20Hygiene%20.pdf

Sleep Foundation. (n.d.). Mental health and sleep. Retrieved from https://www.sleepfoundation.org/mental-health

RAND Europe. (2023). The societal and economic burden of insomnia in adults. Retrieved from https://www.rand.org/randeurope/research/projects/2023/societal-and-economic-burden-of-insomnia.html

Sleep Foundation. (n.d.). Anxiety and sleep. Retrieved from https://www.sleepfoundation.org/mental-health/anxiety-and-sleep

National Center for Biotechnology Information. (2021). Relationship between insomnia and depression in a population-based sample of 7,466 Finns. Retrieved from https://www.ncbi.nlm.nih.gov/pmc/articles/PMC8296753/

U.S. Department of Veterans Affairs. (n.d.). Sleep problems and PTSD. National Center for PTSD. Retrieved from https://www.ptsd.va.gov/understand/related/sleep_problems.asp

Sleep Foundation. (n.d.). Cognitive behavioral therapy for insomnia (CBT-I): An overview. Retrieved from https://www.sleepfoundation.org/insomnia/treatment/cognitive-behavioral-therapy-insomnia

Cleveland Clinic. (n.d.). What is the ideal sleeping temperature for my bedroom? Retrieved from https://health.clevelandclinic.org/what-is-the-ideal-sleeping-temperature-for-my-bedroom

Harvard Health Publishing. (n.d.). Blue light has a dark side. Retrieved from https://www.health.harvard.edu/staying-healthy/blue-light-has-a-dark-side

Healthline. (n.d.). Why a white noise machine may help improve your sleep. Retrieved from https://www.healthline.com/health/sleep/why-white-noise-may-help-you-get-your-best-sleep-ever

Sleep Foundation. (n.d.). How to build a better bedtime routine for adults. Retrieved from https://www.sleepfoundation.org/sleep-hygiene/bedtime-routine-for-adults

Sleep Foundation. (n.d.). The best foods to help you sleep. Retrieved from https://www.sleepfoundation.org/nutrition/food-and-drink-promote-good-nights-sleep

Johns Hopkins Medicine. (n.d.). Exercising for better sleep. Retrieved from https://www.hopkinsmedicine.org/health/wellness-and-prevention/exercising-for-better-sleep

Sleep Foundation. (n.d.). Surprising ways hydration affects your sleep. Retrieved from https://www.sleepfoundation.org/nutrition/hydration-and-sleep

National Center for Complementary and Integrative Health. (n.d.). Melatonin: What you need to know. Retrieved from https://www.nccih.nih.gov/health/melatonin-what-you-need-to-know

Harvard Health Publishing. (2015). Mindfulness meditation helps fight insomnia, improves sleep. Retrieved from https://www.health.harvard.edu/blog/mindfulness-meditation-helps-fight-insomnia-improves-sleep-201502187726

WebMD. (n.d.). Progressive muscle relaxation for stress and insomnia. Retrieved from https://www.webmd.com/sleep-disorders/muscle-relaxation-for-stress-insomnia

National Center for Biotechnology Information. (2017). Tai chi improves sleep quality in healthy adults and older adults with insomnia. Retrieved from https://www.ncbi.nlm.nih.gov/pmc/articles/PMC5570448/

National Center for Biotechnology Information. (2021). Effects of aromatherapy on sleep disorders: A systematic review and meta-analysis. Retrieved from https://www.ncbi.nlm.nih.gov/pmc/articles/PMC8084014/

ScienceDirect. (2022). Effects of cognitive behavioral therapy for insomnia (CBT-I). Retrieved from https://www.sciencedirect.com/science/article/pii/S1087079222000594

WebMD. (n.d.). Keeping a sleep diary. Retrieved from https://www.webmd.com/sleep-disorders/how-to-use-a-sleep-diary

Sleep Foundation. (n.d.). Sleep restriction therapy: Everything you need to know. Retrieved from https://www.sleepfoundation.org/insomnia/treatment/sleep-restriction-therapy

National Center for Biotechnology Information. (2019). Cognitive-behavioral therapy for insomnia: An effective and affordable treatment. Retrieved from https://www.ncbi.nlm.nih.gov/pmc/articles/PMC6796223/

Healthline. (n.d.). Hormonal insomnia: Symptoms, causes, treatments. Retrieved from https://www.healthline.com/health/insomnia/hormonal-insomnia-symptoms

National Center for Biotechnology Information. (2020). Sleep in the elderly. Retrieved from https://www.ncbi.nlm.nih.gov/pmc/articles/PMC7723148/

National Center for Biotechnology Information. (2023). Sleep deprivation, sleep disorders, and chronic disease. Retrieved from https://www.ncbi.nlm.nih.gov/pmc/articles/PMC10487788/

Healthline. (n.d.). Sleep tips for shift workers: How to get the rest you need. Retrieved from https://www.healthline.com/health/healthy-sleep/irregular-schedule-10-tips-to-get-you

Printed in Great Britain
by Amazon